D0322763

THE PHYSICAL CARE OF PEOPLE WITH MENTAL HEALTH PROBLEMS

SAGE has been part of the global academic community since 1965, supporting high quality research and learning that transforms society and our understanding of individuals, groups and cultures. SAGE is the independent, innovative, natural home for authors, editors and societies who share our commitment and passion for the social sciences.

Find out more at: **www.sagepublications.com**

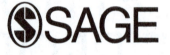

LIS LIBRARY

Date	Fund
10/4/13	mm-Wor

Order No
2389885

University of Chester

Edited by
Eve Collins, Mandy Drake & Maureen Deacon

THE PHYSICAL CARE OF PEOPLE WITH MENTAL HEALTH PROBLEMS

a guide for best practice

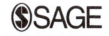

Los Angeles | London | New Delhi
Singapore | Washington DC

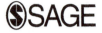

Los Angeles | London | New Delhi
Singapore | Washington DC

SAGE Publications Ltd
1 Oliver's Yard
55 City Road
London EC1Y 1SP

SAGE Publications Inc.
2455 Teller Road
Thousand Oaks, California 91320

SAGE Publications India Pvt Ltd
B 1/I 1 Mohan Cooperative Industrial Area
Mathura Road
New Delhi 110 044

SAGE Publications Asia-Pacific Pte Ltd
3 Church Street
#10-04 Samsung Hub
Singapore 049483

Editor: Susan Worsey
Assistant editor: Emma Milman
Production editor: Katie Forsythe
Copyeditor: Sarah Bury
Marketing manager: Tamara Navaratnam
Cover design: Wendy Scott
Typeset by: C&M Digitals (P) Ltd, Chennai, India
Printed by MPG Books Group, Bodmin, Cornwall

Editorial arrangement © Eve Collins, Mandy Drake and
Maureen Deacon 2013

Chapter 1 © Mandy Drake 2013
Chapters 2 and 5 © Eve Collins 2013
Chapter 3 © Susan Curtis and Sarah Curtis 2013
Chapter 4 © Siobhan Tranter 2013
Chapters 6 and 13 © Maureen Deacon 2013
Chapter 7 © Phil Cooper and Jane Neve 2013
Chapter 8 © Jo Bates 2013
Chapter 9 © Louise Shorney and Richard Shorney 2013
Chapter 10 © Ben Green 2013
Chapter 11 © Clare Street 2013
Chapter 12 © Julie Hughes 2013

Figures 4.1, 4.2, 5.1 and 5.2 © Sandra Casey 2013

First published 2013

Apart from any fair dealing for the purposes of research or
private study, or criticism or review, as permitted under the
Copyright, Designs and Patents Act, 1988, this publication
may be reproduced, stored or transmitted in any form, or
by any means, only with the prior permission in writing of the
publishers, or in the case of reprographic reproduction, in
accordance with the terms of licences issued by the Copyright
Licensing Agency. Enquiries concerning reproduction outside
those terms should be sent to the publishers.

Library of Congress Control Number: 2012940812

British Library Cataloguing in Publication data

A catalogue record for this book is available from
the British Library

ISBN 978-0-85702-920-1
ISBN 978-0-85702-921-8 (pbk)

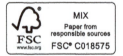

MIX
Paper from
responsible sources
FSC® C018575

CONTENTS

ABOUT THE EDITORS AND CONTRIBUTORS

EDITORS

Eve Collins is the Deputy Head of the Department of Postgraduate Medical, Dental and Interprofessional Education at the University of Chester. As an adult nurse she spent the early part of her career working in critical care before moving into higher education in 2000. Her research and writing interests are best described as eclectic and she developed a special interest in the physical health of individuals with mental health problems following her involvement in delivering educational curricular in this area. The inequitable health and wellbeing of this group inspired Eve's passion to work with her colleagues in mental health to use every opportunity to empower practitioners engaged in the challenging field of mental health practice to support the physical wellbeing of their clients.

Mandy Drake is a Senior Lecturer in Mental Health at the University of Chester. She entered academia 3 years ago following an 18-year career as a mental health nurse and psychological therapist in the community. Prior to joining the university, Mandy worked in primary care and it was here that she started to become interested in the relationship between physical and mental health. Her work in the university has allowed her to develop this interest and, as well as editing this much needed text, Mandy is involved in both teaching and research in this area.

Maureen Deacon is the Head of the Mental Health and Learning Disability Department and Professor of Continuing Professional Development in Health Care at the University of Chester. Maureen's professional background is in mental health nursing, though her first nursing qualification was as a State Registered Nurse and her first job was as a staff nurse in a specialist cancer hospital. Maureen spent the first 20 years of her career in the National Health Service as a practitioner in both inpatient and community settings , as a clinical leader and manager. During this time she was privileged to be supported in doing her first part-time degree in Health Studies at the Manchester Metropolitan University. Much to her surprise (having left school with an A' level in Needlework!) Maureen found higher education to be an incredibly engaging challenge and this experience opened a new career door for her. Pivotal to her student experience was the generous support and critical encouragement of some amazing academics and she hopes that she has done their excellent role modelling some small justice in her own academic career.

Maureen has worked in higher education since 1995 and gained her PhD in 2004: an ethnographic study of acute inpatient mental health nursing. She joined the University of Chester in 2009. Her research interests largely concern real-life health care practice in context. Maureen is interested in how organisational life both shapes and is shaped by nursing work. Her teaching has returned time and again to the relationships between mental and physical health and she was delighted to be invited to share in editing and writing this important book.

CONTRIBUTORS:

Jo Bates has lived and worked in Australia, Canada and the UK. Her specialist area is women's health and sexual health. She has worked as a midwife, Clinical Nurse Specialist in Women's Health and also as a GUM/HIV nurse. Jo is currently working as a Senior Lecturer at the University of Chester in the Department of Midwifery and Reproductive Health.

Phil Cooper is a nurse consultant who has worked in both substance misuse and mental health fields for nearly 20 years. He has developed training programmes regarding mental health substance use and has been instrumental in developing proactive measures to manage substance misuse in acute care mental health settings in the North West of England. Phil has been active in supporting the development of a drop-in group for people with mental health substance use issues and developing a format to assess intoxication levels when people present to mental health services.

Sue Curtis works as a Specialist Diabetes Dietician at Manchester Diabetes Centre, Manchester Royal Infirmary and St Mary's Maternity Hospital. She also develops training courses for staff and patients on diabetes, insulin dose adjustment and weight management. Sue's team has set up a type 2 diabetes education patient steering group to keep patients at the heart of Diabetes Centre plans.

Sarah Curtis is a Trainee Anaesthetist at Leighton Hospital in Crewe. Sarah is enjoying the opportunity to learn the skills required in anaesthetics and is currently particularly interested in orthopaedic anaesthetics

Professor Ben Green is a Consultant Psychiatrist who has published on the psychopharmacology of antipsychotics and antidepressants. He edited the book *Focus on Antipsychotics* in 2004 and has published recently on the psychopharmacology of PTSD. He is Professor of Postgraduate Medical Education and Psychiatry at the University of Chester.

Julie Hughes has worked in infection prevention and control for over 20 years in a wide variety of settings, including general and paediatrics and more recently in mental health and learning disabilities. Her main interests are in educating health care workers around infection prevention and control in this field and what affects their practice and compliance. Julie has recently undertaken a doctorate in this area and is also passionate about service user involvement in infection prevention and control.

Jane Neve is a Nurse Consultant with 5 Boroughs Partnership NHS Foundation Trust, where her focus is the care of individuals with serious mental illness. Jane has worked with this client group in a variety of settings since qualifying as an RMN 23 years ago; her particular interest being psychosocial interventions and the physical health needs of those with SMI. Jane also has an interest in medico-legal issues, particularly negligence, and has completed the academic stages of legal training.

Louise Shorney is a Head of Department in the Faculty of Health and Social Care at the University of Chester where she has worked for the past 6 years. Louise is registered nurse with over 20 years experience. Her areas of interest are tissue viability, orthopaedics and long term conditions. Louise teaches tissue viability to a variety of level of health care workers. Louise has published in numerous peer reviewed journals and has is currently writing a book chapter on wound care for people with mental health conditions. This is a joint collaboration with Richard. She is also registered for a PhD investigating the interpretation and implementation of the role of the community matron.

Richard Shorney is Managing Director of Real Healthcare Solutions. He has over 16 years' experience in clinical and commercial health care settings. Richard has a diverse skill set that has been developed in both clinical practice and through having worked in the health care industry for a blue-chip company. The company Real Healthcare Solutions has been established to utilise Richard's skill set for the benefit of health care organisations, industry, the clinician and ultimately promote and improved cost-effective outcomes for the patient.

Clare Street is a Senior Lecturer in the Department of Nursing at Manchester Metropolitan University, UK. She is Programme Leader for the part-time, BSc (Hons) Contemporary Health Practice degree. Her main interests and teaching responsibilities are around public health, change management and ethics.

Siobhan Tranter is a Lecturer at Bangor University in Wales. She is part of the teaching team on the BSc Nursing and MSc programmes within the university. Siobhan is an active researcher within the department and her interests include the effects of language and culture on health care and the physical health of people with serious mental illness.

ACKNOWLEDGEMENTS

The publishers and authors would like to thank Sandra Casey for the use of the following illustrations:

Figure 4.1 Heart

Figure 4.2 PQRST

Figure 5.1 Lungs

Figure 5.2 Alveoli

1

THE PHYSICAL HEALTH NEEDS OF INDIVIDUALS WITH MENTAL HEALTH PROBLEMS – SETTING THE SCENE

MANDY DRAKE

Learning outcomes

By the end of this chapter you should be able to:

- Identify the main physical health conditions affecting individuals with mental health problems
- Explain the reasons for poor physical health among this client group
- Discuss the barriers to physical health improvement
- Provide an overview of the political agenda in relation to physical and mental health co-morbidity
- Debate the mental health practitioner's role in physical health care

INTRODUCTION

There is growing awareness in clinical practice of what researchers have known for some time, which is that people who experience mental health problems are highly susceptible to physical ill health. This is particularly true of individuals who have a severe mental illness (SMI), such as schizophrenia or bipolar disorder, who are at a significantly increased risk of acquiring a range of physical health conditions (Northrop 2009; Waldrock 2009).

It is not just those with mental health problems who experience physical health conditions; indeed, poor physical health is a growing concern across society as a whole, but of the estimated 17.5 million of the UK population who were living with a chronic physical illness in 2005, the prevalence was much higher where there was a co-morbid mental health problem present (Department of Health 2005b).

While research has consistently shown the poorer physical health of individuals with mental health problems (Phelan et al. 2001), it has been just as consistent in highlighting the neglect of these (Roberts et al. 2007), a neglect some would speculate has contributed significantly to the premature deaths seen in those experiencing a mental health problem.

The shortened life expectancy of this group is a global problem that has been apparent for many years (Nash 2010a). While it could be argued that the heavy focus on suicide prevention in current UK mental health services is an attempt to reverse this, on its own this is ineffective as 60% of premature deaths are as a result of physical health conditions (Brown 1997).

The majority of studies investigating life expectancy have focused on individuals with SMI and early estimates suggested that the presence of a mental illness equated to 10 years of lost life (Newman and Bland 1991). A later study estimated that this had increased to 10–15 years (Richardson and Faulkner 2005), while the most recent suggestion is that people with SMI will die, on average, 25 years earlier than the general population (Parks et al. 2006; Tiihonen et al. 2009). Not only does this corroborate the findings of Saha et al. (2007) that people with SMI are dying at a younger age now than they were 30 years ago, but it is at odds with the majority of the world's population who are enjoying increased longevity (Bradshaw and Pedley 2012).

As well as acknowledging the shocking statistics above, the Coalition government's strategic vision for mental health (Department of Health 2011a) recognises the role poor physical health plays in this, adding that not only is life expectancy of this group vastly reduced, but during their lives individuals with mental health problems will experience far more physical ill health than the general population.

This chapter aims to provide an introduction to the topic of the physical health needs of individuals with mental health problems by presenting an overview of what is currently known. It starts by outlining the main physical health conditions that pose a particular risk to this group before asking why this is. It then discusses what is preventing the health of those with mental health problems from improving before taking a brief look at the UK government's views through recent health policy and guidance. Finally, the role of the mental health practitioner is explored with suggestions from the literature about how this role could become pivotal in the much needed development of physical health care for this vulnerable client group.

THE PHYSICAL HEALTH NEEDS OF INDIVIDUALS WITH MENTAL HEALTH PROBLEMS

CARDIOVASCULAR DISEASE

Cardiovascular disease (CVD) is a collective term for coronary heart disease (CHD), stroke and peripheral vascular disease (Daniels 2002) and there is much evidence to suggest that individuals with mental health problems, particularly those with schizophrenia, are two to three times more likely to experience this than the general population (Brown et al. 2000; Osby et al. 2000).

Of these conditions it is CHD that is the biggest threat to the population's health, as this is now considered the leading cause of death worldwide (Aboderin et al. 2002). However, where one half of all deaths in the population are as a result of CHD, in individuals with SMI it is estimated to be two-thirds (Hennekens et al. 2005), indicating a very significant risk for this group.

METABOLIC SYNDROME

Metabolic syndrome is closely related to CHD in that it encompasses a number of risk factors for heart disease, such as increased blood pressure and obesity, and as such individuals with metabolic syndrome are at an increased risk of developing CHD (Nash 2010a). In addition, though, metabolic syndrome consists of impaired glucose tolerance, insulin resistance and type 2 diabetes (World Health Organization 1999).

While metabolic syndrome as a whole is two to three times more common in individuals with a severe mental illness (McEvoy et al. 2005), it is type 2 diabetes that has received most attention. In particular the relationship between schizophrenia and diabetes has been widely investigated; perhaps more so than any other co-morbid physical and mental health condition (Holt and Peveler 2006). This may be due to the controversy that exists in relation to the part that psychopharmacology may play in contributing to diabetes in this client group, but also as there is no agreement on how prevalent it is.

Robson and Gray (2009) suggest that type 2 diabetes occurs in approximately 15% of people with schizophrenia compared to 5% of the general population, indicating a threefold increased risk. McIntyre et al. (2007), however, propose this could be as high as four to five times that of the general population, increasing the risk even further. Despite the focus of the research being on those with schizophrenia, Robson and Gray (2009) suggest that the risk may actually be higher for individuals with bipolar disorder, but this is still unknown.

Where only 30% of the population with type 2 diabetes are diagnosed under the age of 55, it is 41% for individuals with schizophrenia and co-morbid diabetes, indicating that they develop diabetes at a younger age (Nash 2010a). Furthermore, only 9% of the general population with diabetes have died compared to 23% with SMI, demonstrating that not only do individuals with mental health problems develop diabetes more, and at an earlier age, but that they have a significantly poorer prognosis (Nash 2010a).

RESPIRATORY DISORDERS

During the years of institutionalised mental health care, respiratory diseases such as pneumonia were the major causes of death among its inhabitants (Brown 1997). While this is no longer the case, respiratory disorders among individuals with mental health problems are still high, with asthma, chronic bronchitis and emphysema being more prevalent among this group than the general population (Saha et al. 2007).

Although the exact prevalence of respiratory conditions in individuals with mental problems remains unknown, a US study found that 9% of people with SMI had asthma, 8% emphysema, 20% chronic bronchitis and 23% chronic obstructive pulmonary disease (Himelhoch et al. 2004). The latter, when compared against the 5% prevalence rate in the general population (Himelhoch et al. 2004), demonstrates a markedly increased risk, giving credence to Brown et al.'s (2000) estimate that individuals with mental health problems are four times more likely not only to experience chronic respiratory diseases but to die from them. Once again, the high risk that respiratory disorders present to both the morbidity and mortality of those with mental health problems is very apparent.

CANCER

Cancer presents a more confusing picture with current knowledge being mixed, if not contradictory. The consensus seems to be that there are some forms of cancer that are present more often than expected in individuals with mental health problems (Hippisley-Cox et al. 2007) but, on the whole, rates are similar or even slightly less than those in the general population (Mortensen 1994).

Breast cancer is generally accepted as posing a risk to women with SMI, with one study identifying a 42% increased risk in women with schizophrenia when compared to the general population (Hippisley-Cox et al. 2007). The same study also identified an extremely worrying 90% increased risk of bowel cancer among people with SMI, which the Disability Rights Commission (2007) confirmed in their estimation that individuals with schizophrenia had twice the risk of developing bowel cancer than the general population.

Rates of lung cancer are where most of the current contradiction lies, with Hippisley-Cox et al.'s (2007) study finding a 46% decreased risk in individuals with SMI, suggesting that there may actually be a protective link between the two conditions. Two earlier studies, however, found rates of lung cancer to be twice as high in people with schizophrenia (Brown et al. 2000; Lichtermann et al. 2001), although these were a measurement of mortality, not morbidity.

While the rates of lung cancer may in fact be lower among those with SMI, it may be the case that for those who contract it the death rate is much higher, raising the question of what happens during the progression of this disease that has such a negative impact on the outcome of those with SMI. Before moving on, take some time to think about Action Learning Point 1.1.

Action Learning Point 1.1

Think about the physical health of the clients you work with:

- Which of the conditions outlined do you come across?
- Are these conditions clearly identified in the care plan?
- Do you see physical care carried out?

WHY DO INDIVIDUALS WITH MENTAL HEALTH PROBLEMS HAVE SUCH POOR PHYSICAL HEALTH?

The reasons for the poor physical health of those with mental health problems are complex and varied and the general agreement is that it is a number of interlinking factors that present as a risk. These factors can be separated into health behaviours and treatment.

HEALTH BEHAVIOURS

Many of the conditions outlined are considered to be preventable through lifestyle management but there is widespread opinion that unfortunately individuals with mental health problems expose themselves to adverse lifestyle choices (Wand and Murray 2008). Such choices primarily include high rates of smoking, poor diet and lack of exercise, but co-morbid substance misuse and unsafe sexual practices can be considered among these (Lambert et al. 2003; McCreadie 2003).

Most of us know that the choices we make inevitably impact on our health and we would agree that there is a sense of individual responsibility around these choices. Applying the same level of responsibility to those with mental health problems may not, however, be fair as not all of the above behaviours are choices. Indeed, Robson and Gray (2009) argue that such behaviours may in fact be more accurately seen as the physical, psychological and environmental consequences of having a mental health problem and the treatments that are prescribed for this, and ask that professionals reconsider the use of the term lifestyle choices.

Smoking

Tobacco is the single largest causative factor for lung cancer and respiratory disease and is a contributory factor in both diabetes and cardiovascular disease (Gough and Peveler 2004; Robson and Gray 2007; Nash 2010a). The prevalence of smoking among individuals with mental health problems is known to be high, with estimates of up to 80% in those with SMI (McCreadie 2003), which is three times that of the general population (De Leon et al. 2002). In addition, individuals with SMI are heavier smokers, smoking on average in excess of 23 cigarettes a day (Kelly and McCreadie 2000).

While the negative impact of smoking is clearly outlined, there are also positives, in particular the reduction of psychiatric symptoms through the interaction of nicotine and dopamine (Robson and Gray 2007). Smoking is also ingrained in the very culture of mental health, adding to the challenge of reducing this behaviour.

Diet

The physical health consequences of poor diet include CHD, type 2 diabetes and some forms of cancer, as well as obesity, which in itself presents a risk factor for the conditions discussed (McCreadie 2003; Gough and Peveler 2004; Robson and Gray 2009). Brown et al. (1999) found a diet that is high in fat and low in fibre to be most characteristic of individuals with mental health problems, while McCreadie (2003) found a low intake of fruit and vegetables. In both studies excess weight gain was evident with 86% of women and 70% of men in McCreadie's study being overweight. Similar results were found in a Spanish study where the dietary habits of individuals with mental health problems identified unhealthy foods leading to weight gain (Simonelli-Munoz et al. 2012). Whereas these studies all suggest a diet that is different in content to the general population, this was not the finding of Strassnig et al. (2003), whose American study reported little difference in content but a significant increase in calorie consumption, suggesting that it was the latter that resulted in the observed obesity. It seems, then, that it is both the type and amount of food consumed within the diet of this client group that present a risk and it is both that should therefore be the target of any proposed change.

Exercise

A lack of exercise is a health risk across all of society and in 2003 the World Health Organization (WHO) identified this as one of the leading causes of death in developed countries (WHO 2003a). Not only is a low level of exercise a significant factor in the development of CHD, but it is a contributory factor for diabetes and some forms of cancer (Gough and Peveler 2004; Robson and Gray 2009). Despite the low levels of physical activity across society as a whole, people with mental health problems have been found to have even lower levels of activity, with barriers to increasing this being reported as fatigue, poor confidence and a range of psychiatric symptoms (Ussher et al. 2007).

TREATMENT

Whether the treatments provided for mental health conditions contribute to the development of physical health conditions is a controversial topic, with psychotropic medication being at the centre of this. The link between antipsychotic medication and diabetes has been highlighted for some time (Gough and Peveler 2004; Healy 2009) but whether there is a direct link or whether diabetes occurs as a result of the weight gain that is acknowledged to be a side-effect of the medication is not yet clear.

Psychotropic medication is also associated with CVD, but this again could be as a result of the weight gain as opposed to being more directly linked (Wirshing et al. 2002). As it stands, the current literature by no means offers a conclusion.

As a result of the ambiguity around the effects of medication, many regard psychotropics to be adverse to physical health and, unlike the risks posed by health behaviours, warn that they are a risk that is unique to those with mental health problems (Nash 2010a). While psychotropic medication has a role to play in the physical ill health of this group, Gray (2012) reminds us that there are many other factors at play too and asks that all risk factors be considered for modification, not just medication. Turn your attention now to Action Learning Point 1.2.

Action Learning Point 1.2

Choose a client that you are working with who has a co-morbid physical health condition.

- Identify the health behaviours they have that may be contributing to their poor health.
- Find out what medication they are on and any adverse effects of this.
- Make a list of your client's risk factors in relation to their physical health.

WHAT IS PREVENTING THE PHYSICAL HEALTH OF INDIVIDUALS WITH MENTAL HEALTH PROBLEMS FROM IMPROVING?

As there are reasons for the poor physical health of this client group, there are also reasons for their continued existence as clearly many of the risks are modifiable. These too are multifaceted, but what they have in common is that they act as barriers to the improvement of the current health inequality.

THE MENTAL HEALTH CONDITION

The first barrier is the mental health conditions themselves and the effects of these on the individual's ability to seek help. It has been suggested that people with mental health problems are less likely to report physical symptoms, may in fact be prevented by cognitive deficits from detecting physical problems or may have a high pain tolerance associated with psychotropic medication (Healy 2009; Robson and Gray 2009). In addition, the negative symptoms of psychosis may reduce the ability and motivation of the individual to both seek and engage in behaviour change, thus significantly reducing the chances of effective health improvement.

The majority of barriers, however, relate to the care delivered and whose role this delivery is. The latter is an issue that many mental health practitioners have yet to resolve.

CARE DELIVERY

There is a lot of evidence to suggest that people with mental health problems receive substandard physical health care (Roberts et al. 2007; Lawrence and Kisley 2010). In fact, this poor care was reported by the Disability Rights Commission in 2006 and was reinforced by the Healthcare Commission's (2008) review of Mental Health Trusts, which identified that only 56% of all in-patients had received some form of physical health intervention. A subsequent review in 2011 sought the views of service users themselves, with 37% reporting that they had received no physical health care at all and 33% saying that what they had received was inadequate (Care Quality Commission 2011). It is perhaps not surprising, then, that Robson and Gray (2009) suggest that health care professionals contribute to the poor physical health of those with mental health problems, although they state that this is often subconsciously done and due mainly to a lack of appropriate knowledge and skills, uncoordinated care and inappropriate attitudes.

Lack of knowledge and skills

Several studies have investigated the knowledge and skills of mental health professionals, reaching an overall conclusion that there is indeed a shortfall in relation to physical health (Wand and Murray 2008; Nash 2010a). That is not to say, however, that there is a complete absence of such skills in the workforce; indeed, a review by Blythe and White (2012) found that mental health professionals possessed at least some basic physical health observation skills. Furthermore, Howard and Gamble (2011) report that in their survey of mental health professionals over 80% declared an ability to conduct physical health assessments, monitoring and advice, but unfortunately the same study found little evidence of these actually being carried out.

Uncoordinated care

Uncoordinated care is another potential explanation for the lack of improvement in the physical health of those with mental health problems. Practitioners fail to intervene due to a lack of clarity around their role, which is currently considered indistinct (Chadwick et al. 2012). Not only are practitioners unsure about what care they should be providing, but they are also unclear about who they should refer physical health needs to if they do not intervene themselves. Consequently care is poorly coordinated, leading to service users falling through the net and physical health needs remaining unaddressed (Brown and Smith 2009).

Inappropriate attitudes

Another potential reason is the attitude of the mental health practitioner and what is reported to be a prevailing assumption that individuals with mental health problems are not interested in their physical health needs (Meddings and Perkins 2002). This attitude was noted by the service users in Dean et al.'s (2001) study who refuted the claim, stating instead that their own interest in their physical health had not in fact been mirrored by that of the practitioners. A later study of service users provided reinforcement of all of the above, identifying lack of knowledge and skills, uncoordinated care and inappropriate attitudes as barriers to physical health improvement, although the attitude they referred to concerned 'diagnostic overshadowing' (Chadwick et al. 2012).

Diagnostic overshadowing is a term used to describe the failure of the practitioner to recognise a physical health complaint due to the person's diagnosis of a mental health condition (Jones et al. 2008). In effect, reported physical problems are seen as a symptom of the individual's mental health condition. They are thus disregarded and the literature suggests that this is an attitudinal problem across a number of health professions which leads to inadequate screening and late diagnosis (Disability Rights Commission 2007; Nash 2010a).

Returning to the issue of the mental health practitioner's role, even if this was more clearly defined, there is still the question of whether the practitioner believes this to be their responsibility. This is a topic that researchers have attempted to investigate but there is little consensus as things stand. While most of the practitioners surveyed in the literature agree that physical health needs are important, they also provide reasons for these not to be incorporated into their role.

Blythe and White (2012), for example, identified role ambiguity as a reason that mental health practitioners gave for not taking physical health needs on board, whereas Happell et al. (2012b) report a lack of skills and an unconducive work environment as barriers to engaging in such tasks. A more direct reason found by Hyland et al. (2003) was that mental health practitioners view physical health needs as of secondary importance to those of mental health and Happell et al. (2012b) similarly report the honest assertion that mental health professionals just don't believe that physical health care is a responsibility of their role.

Gray (2012), however, strongly disagrees and, referring to mental health nurses in particular, says that role ambiguity has enabled practitioners to pick and choose favoured aspects of their role for years. He states that the role is very clear; it is about the promotion of a healthy and fulfilling life, and that physical health is as fundamental to this as mental health. While not all will agree with this point of view, Gray is not the only person mooting this. Indeed, the role of the mental health practitioner in the physical health of their clients is something that has been discussed in recent English health care policy, in particular the potential role of the mental health nurse. Before reading about this, take a break and reflect on the questions in Action Learning Point 1.3.

Action Learning Point 1.3

Take some time to think about the following questions. You may want to discuss your thoughts with a colleague or just to reflect on these yourself.

- What knowledge and skills do you have in relation to physical health care?
- How confident do you feel about working with clients' physical health needs?
- Do you think that physical health care is a responsibility of your role?

Perhaps you could raise the last question with your team.

THE IMPACT OF ENGLISH POLICY ON THE PHYSICAL HEALTH AGENDA

Though the focus of this section of the chapter will be on the health agenda within England, no doubt many parallels can be drawn with health policy within other developed countries. Indeed, action learning point 1.4 will ask the reader to consider this. In the meantime, however, a brief overview of the progression of the physical–mental health agenda in England is provided.

It was in 1999 that the first mental health strategy paper was released by the government giving recognition to the debilitating effects of mental health conditions on the population (Department of Health 1999). Mental ill-health was prioritised alongside cancer, CHD and diabetes as major population risks but at the time the interrelationship between mental health and these conditions was not explicit. The need for the physical health of individuals with mental health problems to be incorporated into assessment was, however, identified, though there was no real recognition of the extent of the health inequalities in existence at the time, or of the lack of knowledge in the mental health workforce to address these needs (Hardy and Thomas 2012).

These were recognised some years later; the former in *Choosing Health* (Department of Health 2004a), where both health inequalities and common causes of ill-health were identified. Individuals with mental health problems were again recognised as a group whose health is poorer than the general population and it was reported here that while generally the population was living longer and healthier lives, this was not shared by those with mental health problems. It was also recognised that those with the most severe mental illnesses were prone to considerable weight gain, the link to antipsychotic medication being made. It was similarly noted that the same individuals tended to have poor diets, be obese, smoke more, access health checks less and receive less health promotion.

The need for assistance with this was clearly stipulated and specific guidance was later released to help mental health services implement strategies aimed at improving the physical health of those with mental health problems (Department of Health 2006a). A large focus of this guidance was on developing healthy living initiatives, which, it was suggested, was an ideal role for a mental health nurse.

This was reinforced in the chief nursing officer's (CNO) review of mental health nursing (Department of Health 2006b), which gave a much increased focus on the nurse's role in physical health care. The review emphasises the need for individuals with mental health problems to be viewed holistically rather than as a recipient of treatment for a mental health condition, and states that the underpinning focus of this aspiration should be physical health, which is recognised as a significant risk factor of both morbidity and mortality.

The review further stated that mental health nurses are in a strong position to reduce this risk, making a recommendation that they concentrate on physical health by widening their skills in assessment and in the promotion of physical wellbeing. The skill deficit in the current mental health workforce is, however, acknowledged and advice is given that those nurses already in the workforce should have an assessment of capability and training needs while those who are yet to enter the profession should be socialised to physical health care during their initial training.

The latter has been taken on board in the new standards for pre-registration nursing (Nursing and Midwifery Council 2010). In line with the CNO recommendations, mental health nurses who qualify under the new curriculum will be required to have an in-depth knowledge of common physical health problems, a particular knowledge of those physical health conditions known to be co-morbid with mental health problems, an ability to carry out relevant physical assessments, and adequate knowledge to provide information about physical health treatments and, where relevant, refer on to mainstream services (Nursing and Midwifery Council 2010).

In 2006 and 2009 the National Institute for Health and Clinical Excellence (NICE) produced best practice guidelines for bipolar disorder (2006a) and schizophrenia (2009), which both make explicit suggestions for the incorporation of physical health assessment as part of the overall package of care. While it is recommended that these be conducted in primary care services, there is also acknowledgement that this may not always be feasible and the suggestion is made that mental health practitioners should be ready to take up this responsibility too. Specific consideration in both is given to CVD but incorporating assessment and advice on general wellbeing is also encouraged.

Also in 2009 the National Service Framework (NSF) was superseded by *New Horizons*, the then outgoing government's mental health strategy paper (Department of Health 2009a). The physical health inequity was by this time ingrained in mental health policy but this paper gave specific focus to the need for smoking cessation groups and advised training for all mental health practitioners in order to provide these. The paper was quickly replaced by the Coalition government's mental health strategy (Department of Health 2011a), which also aims to improve the physical health of those with mental health problems. Like the reports before it, the paper identifies the huge inequity that still exists with regard to physical health and sets targets of reducing both the morbidity and mortality associated with these and the mental health population. Specific outcomes that will assist in measuring the success of these include smoking rates, uptake of national screening programmes and rates of admission for alcohol use, all of which are seen currently as risks that need urgent attention.

As can be seen, the UK government has placed a lot of emphasis on reducing the physical health inequalities for individuals with mental health problems yet a recent review of the literature found that very few mental health practitioners had any awareness that such policies and guidelines exist (Blythe and White 2012).

Although there is no statutory obligation for current mental health practitioners to meet the targets of these documents, it is evident that times are changing, certainly in relation to the role of the mental health nurse, which is set to become much more holistic. Physical health care, whether we embrace it or not, will inevitably become part of the role of many practitioners in mental health practice so it is worth considering how the role may develop. First, though, turn your attention to Action Learning Point 1.4.

Action Learning Point 1.4

If you are resident in England:

- Were you aware of the policy guidance available in relation to the physical/mental health co-morbidity?
- What implications do you think it could have on your role and your practice?

If you are not resident in England:

- Are you aware of any policy guidance available on this topic in your country?
- If so, what implications does or could it have on your role and practice?
- If not, think about how you can find out what is available.

THE ROLE OF THE MENTAL HEALTH PRACTITIONER

Robson and Gray (2009) state that the mental health practitioner needs to understand the causes of physical health problems as well as feel confident in assessing, managing and preventing physical ill health.

KNOWLEDGE

When the literature states that there is a skills deficit within the mental health workforce much of it is referring to the lack of knowledge mental health practitioners have generally about the physical health needs of their client group. At the most basic level knowledge of common co-morbidities tends to be poor, but even where this is present there is little knowledge of the signs and symptoms of these

(Wand and Murray 2008). Similarly, knowledge of treatment options and health promotion strategies tend to be largely absent (Bradshaw and Pedley 2012; Happell et al. 2012a).

Wand and Murray (2008) believe that much of the physical morbidity associated with mental health problems is preventable through early recognition of the common occurring disorder, demonstrating the impact that this knowledge could have. Waldrock (2009) further states that having the ability to discuss the potential treatments available can empower individuals to make choices about their own health while knowledge of health promotion can motivate and support them in these choices as well as in improving their overall wellbeing (Hardy and Thomas 2012).

Sufficient breadth of knowledge is therefore crucial to the mental health practitioner role, and for those who are ready to embrace the physical aspect of the role developing this knowledge is a good place to start.

ASSESSMENT

Developing physical assessment skills is also imperative, as was highlighted in the CNO review (Department of Health 2006b), which made a specific recommendation that this become a part of the mental health nurse's role. Indeed, many believe that by simply adapting existing assessment procedures to incorporate physical health the mental health nurse is already ideally placed to take on this function (Gray et al. 2009; Happell et al. 2012b), certainly once the knowledge required has been developed.

Bradshaw and Pedley (2012) suggest that the mental health practitioner should conduct baseline physical tests such as blood pressure, weight and height and that they should monitor these regularly for signs of deterioration. While not in disagreement with this, Tosh et al. (2011) report these to be insufficient on their own and recommend that mental health practitioners make additional assessments. There are a range of physical health assessments that can be carried out by the mental health practitioner to determine the presence of particular conditions but there are also some tools available that are tailored to individuals with mental health problems (Phelan et al. 2004; Shuel et al. 2010), which may present a more usable starting point. Either way, effective physical health assessment is key to improving the overall health status of those with mental health problems and as such is central to the role of the holistic mental health practitioner.

MANAGEMENT

There is no doubt that a large aspect of the mental health practitioner's role when managing physical health conditions is the promotion of a healthier lifestyle, but this is by no means the only aspect. Good coordination of care is essential when working with people with co-morbid conditions as many of these will require expertise that falls outside even the most holistic practitioner's skills. In such an event the role of the mental health practitioner is to facilitate access to the services required and as many practitioners already have the role of care coordinator for their clients, they are in an ideal position to liaise with a range of services (Waldrock 2009), particularly primary care where referral on can be challenging.

As well as facilitating smooth transfer of care, the mental health practitioner has the opportunity to collaborate with the range of specialists that are often available within mental health services, such as dieticians and physiotherapists, developing accessible physical health programmes for their clients (Robson and Gray 2009).

Advocacy is a further area to consider, particularly given the tendency towards diagnostic overshadowing and poor attitudes that have been identified across professional groups. Advocacy can take many forms, from attending appointments with clients to speaking up for their wishes to professional colleagues, and if the physical health needs of individuals with mental health problems are to be taken seriously, Bradshaw and Pedley (2012) believe that advocacy is an essential role.

HEALTH PROMOTION

As both a management and preventative intervention, health promotion is pivotal to the improvement of physical health and thus any role associated with this. While health promotion among mental health staff is currently felt to be poor (Wand and Murray 2008), the adoption of such an approach need not be difficult as even simple behaviour changes can lead to significant health improvements (Happell et al. 2012a).

The focus of the mental health practitioner role should be on modifying lifestyle factors, in particular the encouragement of a balanced diet, with moderation of caffeine and alcohol intake, regular exercise, smoking cessation and, where needed, a weight management programme (Wand and Murray 2008; Bradshaw and Pedley 2012; Hardy and Thomas 2012). Hardy and Thomas (2012) suggest that a good way forward would be to develop health and wellbeing programmes, whereas Robson and Gray (2009) suggest that health promotion should be a routine part of mental care that begins at first contact, thus promoting the centrality of this approach to the mental health practitioner role. Take a look at the final Action Learning Point.

Action Learning Point 1.5

Having read what would be required to incorporate physical health into existing mental health roles, think about the following:

- Is this a role you would like to take on?
- If not, what aspects concern you?
- What knowledge and skills do you need to develop?
- How could you go about developing these?

Why not draw up an action plan and discuss this with your manager?

CONCLUSION

Much of the current focus on mental health services is on the management of risk to patients from suicide; there is no similar concern about the risks from physical ill-health, a risk Bradshaw and Pedley (2012) believe is posed by the lifestyle of individuals with mental health problems and the treatments they are given. While mental health practitioners are in an ideal position to ensure these physical health risks are reduced, they may unfortunately be part of the current problem and a more balanced approach to the mental health practitioner role is being called for where equal importance is placed on physical health.

As has been shown, there is a lot that can be done to improve the poor physical health of those with mental health problems, but only with a change of culture, as the current one supports a view that poor health is inevitable and somebody else's responsibility. Although the adoption of physical health care undoubtedly presents contention and challenge, it also presents opportunity; namely for mental health practitioners to lead the way in the development of integrated and holistic care.

USEFUL RESOURCES

At the time of writing in the UK we recommend the following resources:

Information on policy developments (UK) – www.dh.gov.uk
Health and wellbeing – www.rethink.org
A range of information on physical conditions, screening and treatment – www.patient.co.uk

2

PHYSICAL HEALTH ASSESSMENT IN MENTAL HEALTH PRACTICE

EVE COLLINS

Learning outcomes

By the end of this chapter you should be able to:

- Discuss the importance of providing effective physical health assessments for individuals with mental health problems
- Understand the process of conducting a comprehensive health history
- Identify the health parameters which should be assessed as part of a physical examination for individuals with mental health problems
- Review your own ability to assess your clients' physical health and identify strategies to address any deficits

---

INTRODUCTION

The acquisition of effective assessment skills is at the very heart of clinical competence regardless of the health care profession to which we belong, or the area of practice in which we engage. Yet the term 'assessment' means different things in different contexts. For those of you undertaking an educational programme, 'assessment' may mean the essay or examination by which your knowledge and academic ability will be measured, while in professional practice it is the process of gathering information and data to inform care delivery. Whether we follow the nursing process (see Figure 2.1), the medical model or any other professional service model, assessment is the primary focus of our initial engagement with clients and a vital feature of our ongoing care.

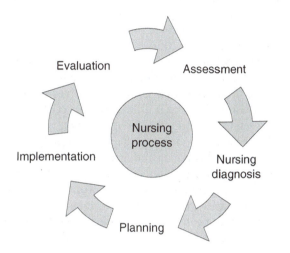

Figure 2.1 The nursing process

This chapter aims to provide mental health professionals with an understanding of the importance of physical health assessments for individuals with mental health problems. However, practical instruction in clinical assessment skills will not be provided and readers are referred to *The Royal Marsden Hospital Manual of Clinical Nursing Procedures* (Dougherty and Lister 2011) or the web-based resources listed at the end of this chapter. The process of conducting a systematic physical assessment will be outlined and practitioners will be encouraged to reflect on their current practice to identify potential areas for improvement.

PHYSICAL HEALTH ASSESSMENT IN MENTAL HEALTH PRACTICE

Well-honed mental health assessment skills are vital tools of the trade for mental health practitioners and act to direct the clinical decision-making process. However, physical health assessment is rarely the primary focus of attention and as such this often poses a challenge for many practitioners.

Early detection of physical disorders such as diabetes, coronary heart disease (CHD) and chronic obstructive pulmonary disease (COPD) is crucial in the facilitation of treatments and interventions which aim to slow the degenerative process, prolonging and enhancing the quality of life of sufferers. Given the hidden morbidity and mortality suffered by those with mental health problems, it should come as no surprise then that the need for more robust methods of assessing their physical well-being has been afforded considerable attention within the literature. Indeed, effective assessment is widely regarded as the first step in addressing the unmet physical health needs of this vulnerable group, leading to frequent calls for mental health professionals to increase their engagement in physical health assessment and care. In the UK, the Department of Health (2006a, 2006b) have made it explicit that there is an expectation that mental health nurses should support and monitor the physical health of people with serious mental illness and facilitate access to appropriate care services should the need arise. In addition, initiatives such as the inclusion of financial remuneration within the General Practitioners (GP) contract (Department of Health 2003) have seen GPs incentivised to offer people with severe mental illness an annual health check. However, at present there is a lack of empirical evidence regarding the effectiveness of this policy and critics point out that it proliferates the system in which care delivery is segregated into physical and mental health care provision. Further, it does little to address the skill deficits among the existing workforce of mental health professionals or to reach those difficult-to-engage clients. Indeed, there is evidence to suggest that professionals engaged in the field of mental health lack both confidence and competence in their ability to assess their clients' physical health.

In 2008 the UK Healthcare Commission found that only 56% of mental health care records indicated that some form of physical health assessment had taken place. This is supported by feedback from mental health clients, 37% of whom reported that they had not been asked about their physical health and 33% expressed the opinion that they had received insufficient support to obtain help with their physical health needs (Care Quality Commission 2011). One explanation for this may be found in the work of Dean et al. (2001) who identified that mental health nurses had a sense of role ambiguity, where they were unsure of their responsibilities in relation to their clients' physical health needs. In 2005 Nash conducted a Training Needs Analysis, with mental health nurses in the UK, and found that although 71% were actively involved in physical health care, only 55% had received any formal training. A staggering 96% of the sample identified a desire for further education regarding physical health assessment skills which goes some way to explain Nash's (2010b) findings that mental health nurses lacked the knowledge required to identify undiagnosed physical disorders. Garden (2005) raises the same concerns about psychiatrists' physical health assessment skills, which Hodgson and Adeyemo (2004) describe as 'variable'.

Clearly there are international variations in the structure of educational programmes for health care professionals, and it seems that the majority of health care curricula do incorporate the skills for conducting physical health assessments. However, those professionals who go on to work in mental health practice may experience a lack of opportunities to regularly engage in this aspect of practice and as a result become deskilled.

This places many professionals in the unenviable position of feeling that they lack some of the skills needed for contemporary practice and necessitates clearer guidance regarding when, how and by whom physical health assessments should be conducted. Further, it is vital that service managers and clinicians work collaboratively to ensure that systematic, proactive assessment processes are embedded into the fabric of the service and supported by organisational protocols.

Action Learning Point 2.1

Review your own practice in relation to your client's physical health and consider the following;

- How confident are you in your ability to conduct physical health assessments?
- Are the physical health assessment of your clients supported by your organisational policies and protocols?

THE ROLE OF THE MENTAL HEALTH PRACTITIONER

There are a number of ways in which mental health professionals can integrate physical health assessments into their practice but the exact nature of the assessment processes you chose to use will be influenced by your professional role, area of specialty and the particular health risks to your clients. For illustrative purposes, this chapter will explore three key ways in which physical health assessment can be embedded in the real world of mental health practice:

- Holistic practice
- Physical health risk assessment tools
- The comprehensive physical health assessment.

HOLISTIC PRACTICE

The first has application for all mental health professionals and emanates from an acceptance of this aspect of your role and a willingness to embrace it. The current situation, in which individuals' physical and mental wellbeing are deemed the responsibility of different care providers, has proved damaging to clients' wellbeing. Thus clients' physical health can be significantly improved if those professionals with whom they have regular contact are attuned to the early signs and symptoms of deteriorating physical wellbeing. A basic understanding of normal and altered physiology, together with the common signs and symptoms of ill-health, are a prerequisite of quality holistic care, and by reading books such as this and undertaking appropriate training opportunities mental health professionals may extend their knowledge of physical assessment and care and utilise this in their daily practice. That is not to say that those engaged in mental health practice should seek to be all things to all people, but rather that they should use their point of contact as an opportunity to identify poor health, promote physical wellbeing and actively encourage their clients to engage with physical health care services when appropriate.

PHYSICAL HEALTH RISK ASSESSMENT TOOLS

The second aspect of physical health assessment in which many of you will engage is commonly driven by national and professional guidelines and forms part of the risk management process. The concepts of 'risk' and 'risk assessment' are very familiar in mental health practice and recent years have seen a proliferation in the number of risk assessment tools utilised by clinicians in all fields of practice. Indeed, in the UK clinical guidelines commonly dictate that some risks are assessed for all clients regardless of diagnosis or location of care, and as a result some practitioners will be accustomed to risk assessing for malnutrition using the Malnutrition Universal Screening Tool (MUST) (NICE 2006c), falls among over-65 year olds (NICE 2004a), and the side-effects of medication (NICE 2002), to name but a few. This is a highly focused method of physical health assessment in which one particular aspect of health is assessed to identify the risk of a negative outcome for the client and expedite preventative measures. However, the risks which fall under the critical gaze of health regulators may well be those of greatest relevance for the general population and are not always reflective of the needs of mental health clients. An example of this is the risk of malnutrition, which is a prominent concern among the acute inpatient population of general hospitals, where many patients have periods of being 'Nil By Mouth' or have ailments which impede their ability to eat, but is less relevant on a mental health secure unit were over-eating or poor dietary choices and obesity are more prevalent problems. This may be a cause of frustration to practitioners who may question the relevance of blanket screening, although I would urge you to utilise such physical health risk assessment tools in conjunction with your clinical judgement and, where possible, to adjust them to suit your client profiles.

Review your practice in relation to these two methods of assessing your clients' physical health by completing Action Learning Point 2.2

Action Learning Point 2.2

Reflect on your own practice and consider the following

- Are you are attuned to the signs and symptoms of physical ill health and do you actively encourage your clients to engage with physical health care services?
- What specific physical risks do you assess for, how appropriate is the risk assessment tool and could it be adapted to better meet the needs of your client group?

THE COMPREHENSIVE PHYSICAL HEALTH ASSESSMENT

The final way in which mental health practitioners can incorporate physical health assessments into their practice involves a more comprehensive means of assessing the physical health risks faced by clients. Recent years have seen sterling efforts made to devise assessment tools to guide mental health professionals with this endeavour. Notably Shuel et al. (2010) offer the Health Improvement Profile (HIP), while Phelan collaborated with Rethink Mental Illness to devise the Physical Health Check (PHC) (Phelan et al. 2004). Both tools aim to elicit a comprehensive range of information regarding the individual's past medical history, lifestyle and contact with physical health care services. A fundamental difference lies in the inclusion of additional objective measures such as blood pathology within the HIP assessment process. This may explain why Shuel et al. (2010) recommend that training is required to support the use of the HIP, whereas the PHC is designed so as to negate the need for specific training. Both tools have been subjected to empirical testing, with Shuel et al. (2010) finding an average of six unmet physical health needs, alongside qualitative evidence that health professionals valued the tool. Phelan et al. (2004) measured the success of the PHC in terms of 65% of people having agreed to one or more physical health interventions. Tosh et al.'s (2010) *Cochrane Review* contends that the current emphasis on physical health screening is unsupported by evidence from sufficiently robust randomised control trials (RCT). However, White et al. (2011) report their intention to conduct an RCT into the efficacy of the HIP which promises to enhance our current understaning of this aspect of contemporary practice.

All comprehensive physical health assessments incorporate two key components, a health history and a physical examination.

TAKING A HEALTH HISTORY

Many commentators point out that a detailed and structured discussion with the individual is the most valuable part of a physical health assessment (Peacock 2004). Indeed, Epstein et al. (2003) suggest that approximately 80% of the information that contributes to a diagnosis is derived during the history-taking process. This should put mental health professionals in a position of strength as they can draw on their communication skills and their existing relationship to engender their client's engagement in this activity.

Taking a comprehensive health history includes consideration of the following: biographical data, past medical history, presenting complaint, lifestyle factors including exposure to health hazards, family history, social history and review of symptoms. Phelan et al. (2004) designed the PHC to be used by community mental health teams; this tool requires a collaborative approach and asks the mental health professional to discuss 27 items divided into four broad sections. The first of these sections covers past medical history, lifestyle and medication (see Box 2.1); the second covers current physical health symptoms; the third considers engagement with physical care services and screening; and the final section incorporates an action plan where the practitioner and client can record any agreed actions deriving from the assessment process.

Box 2.1   General Health and Lifestyle – Rethink Physical Health Check

1   Do you have any diagnosed physical illness or condition? If Yes, please give details: If yes, are you receiving treatment for these? If Yes, please give details:

   List any conditions not currently receiving treatment.

2   Do you have a disability or impairment? If Yes, please give details:

3   Have any of your immediate family or deceased relatives (parents, siblings) had any of the following conditions? Heart disease, Stroke, Cancer, Diabetes, Family history of any other illness/condition. Please specify and give details:

4   Please list all medications you are currently using.
   Do you have any problems with any of these medications (e.g. side-effects)? If Yes, please give details:
   Do you need information about any of the medications you are currently taking? If Yes, please give details:

5   Do you think you eat a healthy diet? (prompts: regular meals, fruit and vegetables, how often takeaways?) Can you give an example of what you eat on a typical day?

6   Do you take part in any physical activity or exercise? (including: walking, cycling, gardening, etc.) If Yes, what do you do? How often do you do this?

7   Do you smoke cigarettes or tobacco? If Yes, how much do you smoke per day? If No, have you smoked in the past? If Yes, please give details:
   Have you tried to stop smoking?
   Do you want to stop smoking? If Yes, is there any sort of help that you would like with this?

8   Do you drink alcohol? If Yes, what and how much do you drink?

9   Are you aware of the recommended maximum units of alcohol per week?

10 Do you use recreational or non-prescribed drugs (e.g. cannabis)? If Yes, what do you use and how often do you use them?

11 Are you aware of the risks of sexually transmitted infection? If No, would you like more information on this?
   Would you like further information on any other sexual health issue? (prompts: pregnancy, contraception, impotence, etc.)

12 Looking back over the questions in this section, do you have any concerns about any of these issues or need any further information? If Yes, please give details:

A comprehensive health history must also include an exploration of any current symptoms, and Seidel et al. (2003) offer the useful mnemonic, 'OLDCART', to assist with this process: Onset, Location, Duration, Characteristics, Associated factors, Relieving factors, Treatment. In addition to its importance in the history-taking process, this approach can provide a valuable structure to ensure that all of the pertinent information is obtained when a client complains about an aspect of their physical health (experiencing pain or feeling dizzy, etc.).

The PHC singles out a small number of symptoms for particular attention based on their indicative value in identifying physical health disorders common among this client group (see Box 2.2).

Box 2.2   Symptom Checklist – Rethink Physical Health Check

Increased thirst

Increased frequency of urination

Breathlessness

Weight gain (unexpected)

Weight loss (unexpected)

Fits/blackouts

Constipation

Sexual dysfunction

Chest pain

Source: Rethink Mental Illness (2012) *My Physical Health*. Available at: www.rethink.org

---

The final aspect of history-taking aims to identify whether the client has undergone any physical health screening or attended routine health checks with the wider multidisciplinary team (family doctor, optician, podiatrist, dentist, etc.). This also presents an opportunity to encourage people to engage in self-examination and to attend routine cancer screening appointments. Now review your learning by considering Action Learning Point 2.3.

Action Learning Point 2.3

- Identify what screening services (mammography, hearing and eye tests etc.) your clients are entitled to. Consider whether you currently ask your clients whether they have attended for screening and how you might encourage them to do so.
- Next time a client reports a physical symptom use the OLDCART mnemonic to guide your discussion of the symptoms and reflect on its effectiveness.

CONDUCTING A PHYSICAL EXAMINATION

Physical examinations rely upon the appropriate gathering and interpreting of objective biological data. The most comprehensive approach involves a detailed head-to-toe examination using the techniques of inspection, percussion, palpation and auscultation to systematically assess the health of the individual's head, ears, eyes, nose, throat, neck, thorax, abdomen, limbs, hands and feet (Baid 2006).

Commonly referred to as a 'general survey', this detailed approach is rarely considered appropriate in mental health practice where physical health assessments are more likely to include the recording of base-line vital signs such as temperature, pulse, blood pressure and respirations (Rushforth et al. 1998). The challenge, then, is to expand on the range of physical health data collected while focusing on those parameters which are most indicative of deteriorating physical wellbeing among this client group.

Inspection is the first phase of the general survey and it starts from the very first moment of contact. This is a vital aspect of the assessment process and is a commonly under-appreciated by practitioners, yet it requires no clinical equipment, is accessible to all and is highly informative. It involves forming an initial impression of the individual, observing the client's general appearance, paying particular attention to their weight and fat distribution, which may indicate metabolic and cardiovascular risk factors. The client's gait, posture and the symmetry of the body may be suggestive of medication side-effects or musculoskeletal disorders. Consideration should also be given to the colour, pigmentation, temperature, moisture content and texture of the skin (Rasmor and Brown 2003) as well as the presence of any rashes, bruises or injuries. Cardiovascular or respiratory insufficiency may be indicated by cyanosis and cold peripheries, discoloured nail beds and oedema, while dehydration would be indicated by a lack of moisture and elasticity in the skin. The inclusion of a body map (see Figure 2.2) within the PHC aims to act as a visual aid to help the practitioner and the client identify and provide a detailed description of any current physical symptoms.

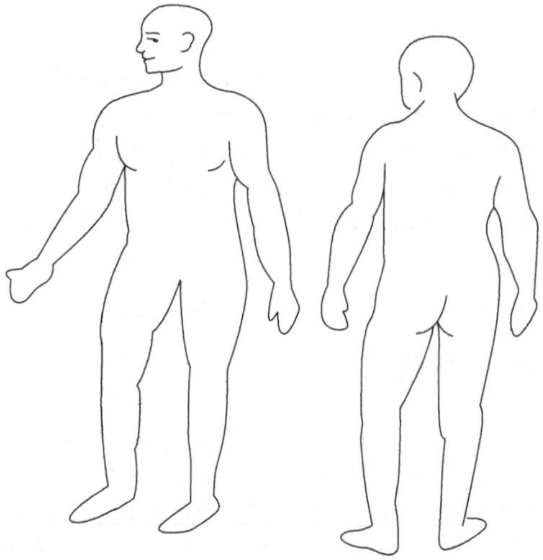

Figure 2.2 Body map rethink

Both the HIP and the PHC recognise the importance of assessing the client's blood pressure (BP), body mass index (BMI), waist measurement and urinalysis. The combined weight of data from these vital signs, reported history and the general survey should afford practitioners a valuable insight into the individual's general wellbeing and can highlight unmet health needs, indicate areas for further investigation or trigger a referral to a physical health care provider. However, White et al. (2009) are not alone in calling for mental health professionals to extend their repertoire of assessment skills as a means of enhancing service provision. They conducted a review of the literature and consulted with experts in the field to generate a list of the key health parameters of specific relevance to those with a mental health problem. Thus, rather than include all of the aspects of a comprehensive general health assessment, the HIP aims to focus on known risk factors for the mentally ill. The final list includes 28 health parameters (see Box 2.2 for some examples) to assess and offers recommended actions should the data fall outside identified parameters. In addition to the parameters already measured, the HIP incorporates an assessment of the client's liver function test and lipid profile, which are widely acknowledged as key risk factors for cardiovascular and metabolic dysfunction, and routine screening is widely advocated in mental health practice. Together with a recording of the pulse and temperature, additional data are also required regarding the client's sleep pattern, caffeine intake, practice of safe sex and attendance at the dentist, optician and podiatrist. The teeth, eyes and feet should be visually inspected to identify any abnormalities.

Given that many mental health professionals are already skilled history-takers and that many of them will be conversant with the means of assessing a client's vital signs, or will have easy access to update these skills, then it is my contention that the process for assessing a client's physical health, outlined above, does not require an extensive programme of clinical skills education. Rather, it calls for a more systematic and focused approach to assessing a client's physical health and an expectation that the information generated will form part of a collaborate plan of care aimed at enhancing the physical wellbeing of the individual. Before moving on, turn your attention to Action Learning Point 2.4.

Action Learning Point 2.4

- Reflect on your current practice and consider which of the health parameters mentioned here are included in your assessment processes; if it would be beneficial to your clients to extend the breadth of assessments how could this be achieved?
- Use the useful resources section of this chapter to review your clinical skills and identify potential opportunities to enhance your repertoire of skills.

CONCLUSION

There is a clear ethical and professional imperative to improve the physical health of the mentally ill and effective physical health assessment could be the first step in realising some meaningful health gains for this vulnerable group. Indeed, the literature indicates that the policy-makers may be justified in championing the application of systematic, proactive assessment processes. As such, service managers and policy-makers must work with the professionals to ensure that they are embedded into the fabric of service and supported by policies, protocols and education. Individual practitioners are also urged to review their own beliefs and practices regarding the physical health of their clients, and to seek appropriate educational opportunities for training and updating skills to enable them to play their part in enhancing this aspect of care delivery.

USEFUL RESOURCES

At the time of writing, in the UK we recommend the following resources:

Skills for Health – www.skillsforhealth.org.uk
Clinical skills – www.clinicalskills.net; www.clinicalskillsonline.com
Physical Health Check – www.rethink.org
Centre for Mental Health – www.centreformentalhealth.org.uk
Royal College of Psychiatry, Improving physical and mental health – www.rcpsych.ac.uk/mentalhealthinfo/improvingphysicalandmh.aspx

3

UNDERSTANDING METABOLIC SYNDROME IN MENTAL HEALTH PRACTICE

SUSAN CURTIS AND SARAH CURTIS

Learning outcomes

By the end of this chapter you should be able to:

- Outline metabolic syndrome and its causative factors
- Discuss the prevalence of the condition in the general population and among individuals with mental health problems
- Examine the progression of metabolic syndrome to type 2 diabetes
- Consider clinical interventions aimed at identifying and managing clients with metabolic syndrome

---

INTRODUCTION

Mental health professionals have increasingly recognised that many of their clients are at an increased risk of weight gain, type 2 diabetes (T2DM) and cardiovascular diseases (CVD), including coronary heart disease (CHD) (Editorial, *The Lancet* 2011). In primary care in recent years there has been a move towards the early identification of risk factors for developing T2DM and CVD, which tend to occur together, and are recognised as 'metabolic syndrome' (Sorrentino 2011). Carmena

(2003) estimates that the prevalence of metabolic syndrome in the general population varies between 11% and 53% across different countries, with increased levels found in western societies and among older age groups. This chapter aims to provide mental health practitioners with an understanding of metabolic syndrome and will consider some of the clinical interventions which have proved effective in its management. Unfortunately, many people with metabolic syndrome do go on to develop CVD and/or T2DM (Shakher and Barnett 2004). While this chapter will explore the progression of the syndrome to T2DM, the reader is referred to Chapter 4 for a detailed exploration of CVD.

METABOLIC SYNDROME

The American Heart Association (www.heart.org) and the National Heart, Lung and Blood Institute (www.nhlbi.nih.gov) define metabolic syndrome as a constellation of interrelated underlying metabolic risk factors that appear to directly cause the development of atherosclerotic cardiovascular disease. Metabolic syndrome has several synonyms: 'insulin resistance syndrome', 'syndrome x' and 'Reaven's Syndrome (Krentz and Bailey 2001). Reaven originally described the syndrome in 1988 and refined it in 1995 (Reaven 1995) to include key features:

- Insulin resistance (defined as decreased insulin-mediated glucose disposal)
- Hyperinsulinaemia (elevated insulin levels in the blood)
- Visceral obesity (increased fat deposits in abdominal organs and fat stores)
- Glucose intolerance (pre-diabetes) or T2DM
- Dyslipidaemia (plasma triglyceride >2.0 mmol/l or HDL – cholesterol <1.0 mmol/l)
- Central obesity (waist circumference >/= 94 cm in men and >/= 80 cm in women)

Expert groups over the years have produced many different definitions. However, simple clinical criteria to diagnose metabolic syndrome are set out in Table 3.1. Three or more of these constitute metabolic syndrome.

Table 3.1 Common physical findings associated with metabolic syndrome

Waist size	>40 inches in men or >35inches in women
Raised triglycerides (fat in the blood)	>/= 150 mg/dl
Low levels of high density lipid (HCL) cholesterol (good cholesterol)	<40 mg/dl in men or <50mg/dl in women
Raised blood pressure	>/= 130/85 mmHg
Raised fasting plasma glucose	>/= 100 mg/dl

Adapted from Grundy et al. (2005)

Source: Grundy, S. M. (2005) 'Metabolic syndrome scientific statement by the American Heart Association and the National Heart, Lung and Blood Institute', *Arterioscl Thromb Vas Biol*, 24: 2243–44.

In 2006 The International Diabetes Federation issued a worldwide definition of metabolic syndrome with general features of: abnormal body fat distribution, insulin resistance, atherogenic dislipidaemia (leading to fatty plaques in blood vessels), elevated blood pressure, proinflammatory (leading to generalised inflammation and endothelial dysfunction) and prothombotic (leading to blood clots) (Alberti et al. 2006).

The management of the disorders clustered in this syndrome, and in the mechanisms involved in its development, is of great interest to researchers who aim to prevent, reduce risk and treat all of these pathologies (Krentz and Bailey 2001). These metabolic changes are predictive of CVD and T2DM (Muntoni and Muntoni 2011) and are highly prevalent among individuals with mental health problems.

METABOLIC SYNDROME IN PEOPLE WITH MENTAL HEALTH PROBLEMS

Compared with the general population, metabolic syndrome is two to three times more common in individuals with severe mental illness (SMI) (McEvoy et al. 2005). People with SMI have nearly twice the risk of dying from CVD, especially at an earlier age (Sukanta et al. 2007). They have a 16–25-year shorter life span primarily due to premature death from CVD (Laursen et al. 2009) and the prevalence of T2DM is four to five times higher in schizophrenia than in the general population (Lund et al. 2001; Newcomer et al. 2002; McIntyre et al. 2007). Generalised anxiety disorder is also positively associated with metabolic syndrome (Knol et al. 2006; Pan et al. 2011). Finally, metabolic syndrome in SMI is a worldwide phenomenon that has been reported in diverse cultures and socio-economic circumstances (Adamson Greene and Rosen 2008). This makes the prevention and management of metabolic syndrome one of the greatest public health challenges of our age.

THE PROGRESSION OF METABOLIC SYNDROME TO T2DM

In order to understand the progression of metabolic syndrome to T2DM knowledge of how the human body metabolises glucose is invaluable.

The central organ involved in glucose metabolism is the pancreas. The pancreas is situated in the abdominal cavity and lies behind the stomach. It has a dual role, a digestive function secreting digestive enzymes (known as pancreatic juice) into the duodenum to break down ingested fats and an endocrine function producing hormones which enable the body to regulate blood glucose levels. The normal blood glucose range is between 3.5 and 5.5 mmols/l before meals and less than 8mmols/l after meals (www.diabetes.org.uk), and deranged blood glucose levels have a detrimental effect on human physiological functioning. The hormones directly involved in the homeostasis of glucose are insulin and glucagon. However, other hormones are also involved, as discussed by Aronoff et al. (2004).

When we ingest carbohydrates in our diet they are broken down in the digestive system and absorbed into the blood as glucose (Colagiuri et al. 1997). This elevates the blood glucose level and stimulates the pancreas to release insulin into the blood stream. The insulin acts like a key and enables the glucose to enter the cells of the body and be used for energy. Insulin also enables the liver to store any excess glucose as glycogen. When the blood glucose level falls, between meals and during the night, insulin production is decreased. At the same time the secretion of glucagon increases. This hormone enables the liver to convert the stored glycogen back into glucose and be released into the bloodstream. In this way the two hormones work together to maintain stable blood glucose levels, providing a steady supply of fuel for the body's cells (Krentz and Bailey 2001).

T2DM is a progressive condition in which the pancreas produces insufficient insulin, the cells become less receptive to the insulin produced (known as insulin resistance) or both. Insulin resistance can occur up to 10 years before T2DM develops, is sometimes referred to as pre-diabetes or impaired glucose intolerance, and is known to affect about 15% of adults from epidemiological studies in North America, Europe and Asia. Of those with pre-diabetes, it is estimated that between 5% and 12% develop type 2 diabetes annually (Diabetes UK 2009).

Over time elevated blood glucose levels damage the cardiovascular system, leading to the build-up of fat and cholesterol inside the vessels. This obstructs the flow of blood, increasing the risk of heart attacks, strokes and causing CVDs such as diabetic ulcers and diabetic retinopathy (retinal damage caused by poor blood supply).

WHAT CAUSES METABOLIC SYNDROME?

While the risk of developing metabolic syndrome increases as we age, there is a wide array of additional risk factors.

LIFESTYLE FACTORS

The effect of lifestyle on physical wellbeing is the subject of a vast amount of research and there is clear and indisputable evidence that lifestyle factors influence both whether the individual develops metabolic syndrome and whether this progresses to CVD and/or T2DM. In particular, the impact of diet, exercise and weight management cannot be underestimated and thus warrant further attention.

Kouki et al. (2011) found that, after genetic inheritance, physical activity level was perhaps the single most important factor influencing the development of metabolic syndrome. Gorczynski and Faulkner (2010) are among a number of researchers who indicate that, compared with the general population, individuals with mental health problems are more likely to be sedentary. As such, this may go some way to explaining the elevated rates of metabolic syndrome among this vulnerable group.

A diet rich in saturated fat (e.g. sausages, fatty meats and cheeses, butter and ghee), trans fats (pies, pastries, deep fried foods and biscuits), and sodium in convenience meals, plus alcohol above recommended limits, individually and synergistically raise the risk of developing cardiovascular disease, in people genetically susceptible to developing metabolic syndrome. Several studies have shown that individuals with mental health problems commonly make poor dietary choices, characterised by limited fruit and vegetables and high fat content (McCreadie 2003).

There is evidence to suggest that dietary combinations such as the Mediterranean-style diet (Esposito et al. 2004), or dietary approaches to prevent and treat hypertension (Azadbakht et al. 2005), are associated with a reduced prevalence of metabolic syndrome and its features. Further, Ruidavets et al. (2007) found that a diet high in vegetables, salad, fruit, berries, whole grains, nuts and fresh or unprocessed frozen fish, and lower-fat dairy products have also been shown by to be protective against developing metabolic syndrome.

Poor diet and sedentary lifestyles also increase the likelihood of obesity. Intra-abdominal obesity tends to cause insulin resistance and as the individual becomes less active, gains more weight or ages, the insulin resistance increases and plasma glucose levels begin to rise, leading to pre-diabetes. A randomised controlled trial by Orchard et al. (2005) indicates that pre-diabetes can be delayed or even reversed if people become more active, eat healthily and lose weight.

It is important to recognise that diet and exercise are not the only lifestyle factors which are predictive of poor physical health. Indeed, many individuals with mental health problems encounter social problems that include long-term unemployment, poverty and homelessness or inappropriate housing. These biological, psychological and socio-economic problems limit choices for healthy food very much among people with SMI, tending to lead to use of ready-meals and takeaways. It is difficult for them to take up exercise opportunities which cost money or involve social situations.

PSYCHOTROPIC DRUGS

Allison et al. (2009) demonstrated that there is clear evidence of psychotropic drugs, including antipsychotics, antidepressants and mood-stabilising medications, being associated with the features of metabolic syndrome and its outcomes of CVD and T2DM. De Hert et al. (2009) presented a comprehensive review of the relationship between types and individual antipsychotic drugs and the features of metabolic syndrome. However, Tiihonen et al. (2009) in an 11-year, population-based cohort study followed up patients with schizophrenia and found that those on long-term second-generation antipsychotic agents (SGAs) had lower all-cause mortality than their untreated counterparts.

Of the antipsychotic drugs, some of the SGAs (also known as atypical antipsychotic drugs) are significantly associated with metabolic syndrome as compared to the first-generation antipsychotics (FGAs) or classical antipsychotic drugs. Of the SGAs, Adamson Greene and Rosen (2008) have deduced that clozapine and olanzapine are the worst offenders by far, with weight gains of 6–7 kg over a few weeks to months, followed by risperidone and quetiapine, whereas aripiprazole and ziprasidone appear to be weight neutral. Although psychotropic drugs are thought to produce metabolic side-effects through weight gain, it has been shown that 25% of patients who had metabolic syndrome did not gain weight. This indicates that these drugs may be producing some of their metabolic effects by direct action on other features such as hypertension and dyslipidemia.

Andersohn et al. (2009) found that antidepressants continue to be implicated with features of the metabolic syndrome, especially amitriptyline (among the old tricyclics) and paroxetine and mirtazapine (among the new generation of serotonin-specific uptake inhibitors), particularly for patients taking these drugs for over two years. Zimmerman et al. (2003), in their review of epidemiology, implications and mechanisms underlying drug-induced weight gain in psychiatric patients, found the so-called mood stabilisers (lithium and valproate sodium) also to be implicated in weight gain.

GENETICS

Some causative factors for metabolic syndrome fall outside the individual's control and vast numbers of individuals around the world have an inherited tendency towards developing T2DM. To date, 38 different genes have been identified as involved in the development of T2DM. Thus some people who have relatively healthy lifestyles and are not obese (BMI < 30) still have insulin resistance. Further evidence of a genetic link for T2DM can be found in the increased prevalence of T2DM among those with a diabetic parent, parents, first- or second-degree relative. The prevalence of diabetes also varies across different ethnic groups with higher levels among people of South Asian or black Caribbean ethnicity.

In addition, genetics plays a part in body fat distribution and individuals who are genetically inclined to have a fat distribution pattern known as an 'apple shape' with fat deposited on the abdomen, chest, upper trunk, back, neck and face are at greater risk of developing metabolic syndrome. This genetically predetermined pattern of fat distribution can be contrasted with a 'pear shape' where fat is deposited on the bottom, hips and thighs.

Further, there is a significant body of literature which supports the idea that people with SMI have an innate propensity to develop metabolic syndrome. This implies a genetic or inherited component, but does not exclude the effects of lifestyle, environment and stress, which are believed to influence the expression of these genes at different stages of the lifecycle. There was some anecdotal evidence for a relationship between SMI and metabolic syndrome before the introduction of antipsychotic drugs, which began in 1952, with the introduction of chlorpromazine in France. A 1944 study of veterans with schizophrenia suggested that some psycho-neuro-endocrine factors linked diabetes and schizophrenia. Raphael and Parsons (1921) found increased glycosuria (glucose in the urine) in people with schizophrenia, which we now know to be suggestive of blood glucose above 10 mmoles/l (pre-diabetes or undiagnosed type 2 diabetes). Similar findings were replicated several times before the introduction and use of antipsychotic medication.

More recently, compared with matched controls (for age, ethnicity, activity level, diet, smoking, and alcohol intake), people diagnosed with their first episode of schizophrenia, and without any exposure to psychotropic drugs, had a significantly higher rates of impaired fasting glucose levels, more insulin resistance, higher cortisol levels, higher adrenocorticotropin (ACTH) levels, and over-activity of the hypothalamic–pituitary–adrenal (HPA) axis function. Ballon and Fernandez (2008) suggested that this deregulation of the HPA axis function was a possible causative factor in loss of blood glucose control. Indeed, there is now biological evidence of metabolic dysfunction in schizophrenia. Nimwegen et al. (2008) found that people with schizophrenia and schizoaffective disorder unexposed to antipsychotic medication, showed more hepatic (liver) insulin resistance compared with matched controls. This was after controlling for differences in intra-abdominal fat mass and other relevant factors. This clearly suggests a direct genetic link between schizophrenia and insulin resistance.

In the case of other mental illnesses, Babić et al. (2010) have concluded that there is abnormal metabolic activity in bipolar disorders. Furthermore, Wolkowitz et al. (2010) have likened long-term depression to a state of 'accelerated aging', because depressed individuals have a higher incidence of various diseases of aging, including metabolic syndrome, cardiovascular, cerebrovascular diseases, and dementia.

While the debate regarding the causes of metabolic syndrome continues, it would seem that mental illness can trigger a pathogenic cycle of disorder, lifestyle, and psychotropic drugs, whereby all the factors associated with the disease lead to the development of the condition. Thus metabolic syndrome and subsequent T2DM look set to continue to impede the physical wellbeing of substantial numbers of people with a mental health problem.

THE ROLE OF THE MENTAL HEALTH PRACTITIONER

Appropriate awareness, knowledge and experience of metabolic syndrome leading to T2DM are a prerequisite of quality holistic care for people with mental health problems. Treatment approaches focus on physical health assessment (explored further in Chapter 2), lifestyle and health promotion strategies (explored further in Chapter 11), and effective care of the diabetic client.

PHYSICAL HEALTH ASSESSMENT

Early identification of the physiological changes which represent metabolic syndrome is a fundamental way in which we can slow the trajectory of the syndrome towards the development of irreversible and life-limiting diseases. Thus all mental health professionals should incorporate physical health assessments into their care. Inexpensive tests such as urinalysis are highly effective in detecting glycosuria (glucose in the urine), which is a key indicator of metabolic syndrome. Weight measurements, blood pressure and blood lipids all offer an insight into the physical wellbeing of clients and should form part of a systematic approach to physical health assessment (as discussed in Chapter 2). Mental health professionals should also have an awareness of the common signs and symptoms of T2DM which Diabetes UK (www.diabetes.org.uk) suggests include:

- going to the loo all the time to pass urine
- feeling very thirsty and drinking a lot
- feeling very tired
- losing weight (and you don't know why)
- regular episodes of thrush or genital itching
- blurred vision
- slow healing of cuts and grazes

The following tests offer a more specific means of identifying metabolic syndrome:

- A fasting blood glucose measurement. In impaired fasting glucose (IFG) the fasting glucose level is raised and is between 6.1 and 6.9 mmols/l. It is thought that one in four adults may have IFG.
- A glucose tolerance test, where blood glucose is measured, then the patient takes a drink containing 75 g glucose, and blood glucose is measured again two hours later. In impaired glucose tolerance and two hours after having the glucose drink, blood glucose level is raised to between 7.8 and 11.7 mmols/l.

Now take some time to consider Action Learning Point 3.1.

Action Learning Point 3.1

Consider the physical health assessment process you utilise in practice.

- How do you identify whether your clients have metabolic syndrome and/or diabetes?
- How effective is this process?
- If it is not effective, consider what adaptations can be made to enhance it?

HEALTH PROMOTION

The aim of health promotion strategies are that the individual is encouraged and supported to:
- become more physically active
- eat a healthy diet, including moderation with alcohol

- lose weight to reduce central obesity and waist circumference
- have sufficient sleep and relaxation

The healthy lifestyle weight loss approach recommended here is fully discussed within the National Institute for Health and Clinical Excellence (2006b) guidance on obesity. Basically, it involves using a 'health trainer approach', getting alongside the person, using open questions and a friendly low-key discussion style to understand their situation and perspectives and gauge their position on the 'cycle of behaviour change'. You also need to assess the person's self-confidence and self-esteem and readiness for change. If the person does wish to try to make some changes, then you should gain a fuller appreciation of the person's situation and support them in developing their own plan for lifestyle change, based on small, achievable steps. You need to discuss any ambivalence about change, and difficulties the person sees as well as the positive aspects and benefits of healthy living. People who initially feel unsure about trying to make change can be encouraged by your interest and be 'contemplative', considering change for the next time you see them.

There is now strong evidence from randomised controlled trials that lifestyle interventions incorporating diet and physical activity can prevent T2DM in high-risk individuals from different ethnic backgrounds, and that intensive lifestyle interventions are rated as very cost-effective. In April 2011 Diabetes UK published evidence-based nutrition guidelines for the prevention and management of diabetes, which offer a rich source of research in the field. Nutrition management has shifted from a prescriptive 'one size fits all' approach to a person-centred approach. The guidelines stipulate that a registered dietician knowledgeable about diabetes care should be providing nutrition advice to all people with diabetes or at high risk of developing diabetes. It is important that people with mental illness who fall into these groups can access a dietician, either via primary care or via their mental health team. The prevention of T2DM is an important aim for anyone with a SMI. The Diabetes UK (2011b) guidelines offer the following advice:

- Weight loss is the most important predictor of risk reduction; loss of at least 5–7% of body weight is effective for prevention.
- Lifestyle interventions including energy restriction, high carbohydrate low-fat diets and increased physical activity can reduce risk; there is no evidence for the most effective dietary approach to achieve weight loss and prevention. Interventions promoting diet alone, increased physical activity alone or a combination are equally effective in reducing risk.
- Dietary patterns characterised by low intakes of saturated fat and higher intakes of unsaturated fat are protective.
- Diets of low glycaemic index/load and higher in dietary fibre and wholegrain are protective.
- Some specific foods (low-fat dairy foods, green leafy vegetables, coffee and moderate intakes of alcohol) are associated with reduced risk.
- Other foods (red meats, processed meat products and fried potatoes) are associated with increased risk.

In practical terms this means eating a varied diet, with regular meals across the person's active 'day', and using low-fat cooking methods. Therefore mental health practitioners need to consider the following when working with their clients:

- Nutrition labelling – food packaging can be very useful provided the consumer under-stands it. Not everyone looks at nutrition labelling, but the health practitioner should enquire about this and be prepared to spend time teaching how to interpret information. There is no international nutrition labelling agreement, but the most common way of showing information is as nutrients per 100 g of food, or per portion, and in comparison with average guideline daily amounts. Traffic guide nutrition labelling, identifying healthy amounts of fat and saturated fat, salt and sodium, calories and sugar content in that food is also often used and is particularly helpful.
- Balanced diet – the Eatwell Plate from the Department of Health (2006a) (see Figure 3.1) has international appeal as a teaching aid for a healthy balanced diet. It illustrates the Eatwell Plate with captions showing the five food groups, and the relative proportions of each food group on the plate to achieve good-quality nutrition and assist weight management.
- Cooking methods – this is really important, as 1 g of pure fat or oil provides 9 kilo calories. People often need advice regarding low-fat cooking methods, so it is important to find out how they cook – fry, boil, etc.
- Portion size – you may also need to explore the volume of food your client eats. One prac-tical way of doing this is to encourage them to show you, using their hands. Our hands in general are in proportion to our body size. Use your own hands, say, to describe a portion of fish (upturn your hand, palm up and keep thumb next to palm). Then make sure they use their own hands to show you their portion sizes. Weight management can be helped by reducing portions of starchy foods by a third or a quarter, if these seem excessive.
- Speed of eating – this is an important part of weight control as the appetite centre in the brain does not receive the message that the stomach is full until 10 to 15 minutes after fullness occurs.

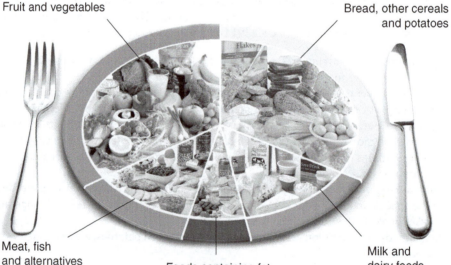

Fruit and vegetables

Bread, other cereals and potatoes

Meat, fish and alternatives

Foods containing fat
Foods containing sugar

Milk and dairy foods

Figure 3.1   The Eatwell Plate (Department of Health 2006a)

The evidence suggests that the most effective way to make and sustain changes is to implement these in incremental steps and, as such, it is advisable to encourage your clients to make one or two changes at a time. Reflect on your learning by considering Action Learning Point 3.2.

Action Learning Point 3.2

Reflect on your own eating and habits and consider the following:

- When you have attempted to implement changes to your diet how easy did you find it?
- What barriers did you encounter?
- What strategies did you use to overcome these barriers and maintain your progress?

Recent years have seen the development of health promotion programmes that combine exercise and dietary change specifically aimed at those with a mental health problem. Faulkner et al. (2010) published a Cochrane review of five small trials where a cognitive or behavioural approach had been used to encourage healthier eating and more physical activity. Two of these had shown a mean weight loss of 3.4 kg. Their guidance for future interventions was:

- Begin weight management close to the diagnosis of the SMI
- Keep dietary changes simple and look at the food environment too
- Aim for gradual increase in physical activity – initially to interrupt continuous sedentary behaviour, with short periods of movement

Very interestingly, Gorczynski and Faulkner (2010) also published a Cochrane review selecting three small randomised trials of people with schizophrenia. Overall, these studies showed that exercise therapy can have a positive impact on mental state and general functioning with no adverse effects, and a limited effect only on physical health outcomes without any changes in weight.

Table 3.2 summarises the 'In SHAPE' individualised health promotion intervention pilot scheme (Van Citters et al. 2010). The intervention was provided by fitness trainers known as 'health mentors' trained in goal setting, motivational interviewing and healthy eating behaviours. Participants included a broad spectrum of individuals with SMI, but excluding people with dementia.

Dropout rates on such programmes can be high and where health resources are limited it is essential to assess readiness for change and consider incorporating motivational strategies. Then those contemplating change can be directed and supported towards free or low-cost community schemes that encourage healthy living. Take a look at Action Learning Point 3.3.

Table 3.2   In SHAPE pilot scheme

Step 1	Assessment (conducted by the health mentor). To include: Physical health assessment. Fitness status and personal fitness goals. Dietary behaviours. Current exercise and preference for type of exercise and setting.
Step 2	Planning (devised in collaboration between the client and health mentor). Individualised fitness plan. Individualised diet plan.
Step 3	Individual fitness instruction and exercise activities (consider cost and access free facilities if possible). Weekly support (provided by the fitness mentor). Group-based activities to support recognition of achievements and education regarding fitness and healthy eating. Ongoing physical health evaluation.

Action Learning Point 3.3

Consider the ways in which you could promote a healthier lifestyle for your clients.

- What challenges and barriers might they face?
- How could you help them to overcome these barriers?

CARE OF THE DIABETIC CLIENT

Upon diagnosis with T2DM, individuals should be assessed by their primary health care team and encouraged, with support, to make any lifestyle changes necessary for them. This may include at the outset beginning to take medication at specified times, gradually making some dietary changes and becoming more active. It is not usually advised that people try to make lots of changes at once. Stopping smoking is usually seen as something to work on later, when the diagnosis has been accepted and the initial anxiety associated with it has subsided somewhat. While people with diabetes can usually drink alcohol within the usual limits set for everyone, some people with high intakes or binge drinking will need support with reducing their intake. Education and support should be tailored to the individual and done gradually. For those with a mental health problem, they have the additional complexity of their co-morbidity and they especially will require guidance, support and understanding.

Health education plays a key part in helping clients gain an understanding of their condition and how to manage it themselves. However, they will need professional support and should be referred to their family doctor or their practice nurse, who may be their key diabetes health professional. They are likely to refer the person to a community dietician who will also prove invaluable, and where possible clients should be given the opportunity to engage in group education about diabetes.

There are various accredited and NICE-approved educational support courses available which offer a structured patient education programme to help people, both newly diagnosed or with established T2DM, better manage their condition. One example of this is the X-PERT patient programme which is based on principles of adult learning (Ewles and Simnett 2003) and is interactive. The programme is facilitated for small groups of individuals and involves participants in making plans and setting goals for change over a series of six sessions, as outlined in Table 3.3.

Table 3.3 The X-PERT patient programme

Week	Title	Content
1	What is diabetes?	Digestion and blood glucose. Healthy lifestyle for looking after diabetes. Understanding your own health measurements (BMI, cholesterol, trigylcerides, HbA1c, blood pressure, albumin: reatinine ratio).
2	Healthy eating with the 'Eatwell Plate'	Energy balance. The benefits of physical activity. Weight management using a 500 calorie deficit. How to assess your own diet.
3	Carbohydrate – an important nutrient in diabetes	What are carbohydrate (starchy and sugary) foods? The amount and type of carbohydrate foods. What carbohydrates are you having?
4	Reading and understanding food labels	Shopping for foods. Looking at the foods you buy. Understanding the traffic light system, guideline daily amounts (GDAs) and nutritional labels.
5	Low and high blood glucose levels	Possible complications of diabetes. Prevention of complications of diabetes. Importance of regular check-ups. Living with diabetes.
6	X-PERT Game	Questions and answers. Comments and feedback. How to continue.

In 2011 X-PERT reported the biggest audit of its outcomes using the national X-PERT database (Deakin 2011). All participating organisations had demonstrated an improvement in blood glucose control and the majority were also demonstrating clinically meaningful improvements to body weight, blood pressure and lipid outcomes by six months.

Medication management is also a fundamental part of effective diabetic care and blood glucose lowering medications fall into three categories: oral hypoglycaemic drugs (tablets), incretin injections and insulin injections. The natural history of T2DM is of a gradual deterioration of pancreatic function and increasing insulin resistance, resulting in an increase of medication. Many types of diabetes tablets work well in combination. The National Institute for Health and Clinical Excellence (NICE) regularly updates guidance on the use of diabetes medications in T2DM, from diagnosis and during progression of the disease (National Institute for Health and Clinical Excellence 2011a). Many people with T2DM do eventually require insulin, although increasing use of incretin injections earlier in the progression of the disease is gradually changing this picture. Table 3.4 lists these with a simple indication of how they work. Medication concordance can be a problematic aspect of diabetes care as people may sometimes refuse to take their diabetes medications, or all medications. Alternatively,

Table 3.4   Common medications for diabetes

Type of medication	Drug name	Mechanism of action
Oral hypoglycaemic drugs	Biguanide – Metformin (Glucophage)	This works by reducing the amount of glucose produced by the liver and increasing the uptake of glucose by the cells of the body. Can reduce appetite a little; does not cause hypoglycaemia (hypo).
	Sulphonylureas – Gliclazide and Glipizide	These work by stimulating release of insulin from the pancreas and are most effective in the early years following diagnosis. Can cause hypoglycaemia.
	Glitazone (thiazolidenedione) – Pioglitazone	Helps to reduce insulin resistance and make the person more sensitive to their own insulin. These require liver function tests to be carried out.
	Meglitinides – Repaglinide and nateglinide	Stimulate insulin release as blood glucose rises, following a meal. These are less likely to cause hypo than sulphonylureas.
	Acarbose	This works by blocking an enzyme in the bowel and delays absorption of dietary starch and sugar. It has a small glucose lowering effect and can cause flatulence.
	DPP–IV (dipeptyl peptidase –IV) inhibitors (gliptins or incretin enhancers) – Sitagliptin and vildagliptin	These work by enhancing the effects of 'incretins', natural hormones produced in the gut after eating. Do not cause hypo and are taken only once daily.

Type of medication	Drug name	Mechanism of action
Incretin injections	Incretins – GLP 1 (Glucagon – like peptide -1) agonists – exenatide and liraglutide	These are based on a human gut hormone. They stimulate insulin secretion, slow emptying of the stomach, inhibit glucose production from the liver and suppress appetite and can facilitate weight loss in motivated people.
Insulin injections	Long-acting analogue – e.g. Lantus and Levemir	Provide additional insulin as steadily released active insulin across 20–24 hours. Daily or twice daily injections. Dose titrated gradually.
	Medium and long-acting insulins, e.g. Insulatard and Humulin I	Provide active changing insulin profile across 12 and 8 hours respectively.
	Short-acting insulins/ neutral insulin, e.g. Insuman Rapid and Actrapid	Provide peak duration of insulin activity over 4 and 3 hours respectively.
	Mixed insulins, e.g. Humulin M3 and Insuman Comb 50	Provide biphasic insulin: mixture of short and longer activity insulin. Injected twice or sometimes three times daily.
	Rapid acting analgues, e.g. Apidra and Humalog	Almost immediate onset of activity after injecting, short duration of activity 2 to 3 hours only respectively.
	Analogues mixtures, e.g. Novomix 30 and Humalogue mix 25	Almost immediate onset of activity after injecting and tapering activity over 8 hours.

they may just decide to stop taking some of them, perhaps worried about side-effects or blaming one medication for how they feel, without a full understanding of what is happening. In general, in T2DM blood glucose levels will tend to rise gradually over a few days. As such, failure to comply with medication and treatment regimes may result in poor glucose control and have a negative effect of the individual's health over the moderate to longer term, but it is unlikely to result in an immediate medical emergency. It is much more serious if people with type 1 diabetes refuse to take their insulin and the diabetes team should be contacted straight away and medical attention sought.

Central to effective care of diabetic individuals is effective liaison among the multi-disciplinary team. Routine health screening is vital to identify the early signs of impairment which can result from diabetes and in particular diabetic clients should be referred to the optometrist for retinal screening and the podiatry service foot screening service.

Before moving on, review your understanding of the care of an individual with diabetes, by considering the following case study.

Derek

You have a new client, Derek, 48 years old, who has schizophrenia and is unemployed, living in a large community residential home where meals are provided. He is single and his extended family lives about 150 miles away. Derek has T2DM which is treated with a single daily injection of Lantus (24 hour background insulin), a single daily injection of liraglutide (Victoza a GLP-1 agonist) and twice daily gliclazide (a sulphonylurea). Derek does have a choice of when he can inject his once daily Lantus insulin and Victoza. He is responsible for his own medications and has aripiprazole and lithium to treat his schizophrenia. Since he began insulin about six weeks ago his very poor blood glucose control is much improved, he has gained 4.5 kg and his BMI is now 34. Derek tends to have periods where he regularly monitors his blood glucose, as advised. He is very capable of home blood glucose monitoring; however, at present he finds it difficult to sustain his motivation for this and for healthy eating and physical activity, although he continues usually to be compliant with his medications, both tablets and injections. Derek attends the local Diabetes Centre and you wish to try to encourage him to eat healthily and become more active.

Please discuss the following questions working individually, in pairs or small groups.

1 How will you gain understanding of Derek's situation and lifestyle?
2 How can you support Derek in preventing relapse into old behaviours?
3 What strategies can you implement to enhance Derek's wellbeing?

Answer guidance:

1 NICE (NICE and National Collaboration Centre for Primary Care 2006) recommends a health trainer approach, using open questions and informal discussion to better understand how clients perceive their health and the options to manage this. In relation to Derek's case, the discussion will focus on his recent weight increase and his management of his diabetes, taking into account his current lifestyle choices. Such discussions will also facilitate exploration of Derek's readiness to change his current lifestyle within the options he has available, given his housing and financial situation, and the 'cycle of change' assisting with this. You can further consider his feelings of self-efficacy.
2 It could be useful to establish a 'baseline' of Derek's current behaviours with respect to diet, physical activity, blood glucose testing and medications. This could then be shared in a joint appointment with Derek's key worker at the Diabetes Centre. Then you can clarify and agree a lifestyle approach and suitable amount of monitoring for Derek to use and plan how you can help him achieve this.
3 You need to be aware of the signs and symptoms of T2DM in order to monitor any potential deterioration. Forming a link with his residential care provider and knowledge of the menu choices from the chef and/or manager to help Derek identify healthy choices he likes or any barriers towards his uptake of these could be explored.

Routine retinal and foot screening is recommended for individuals with diabetes and you can encourage Derek to attend these appointments and also liaise in relation to arranging these.

There are a number of health promotion strategies that you could implement with Derek to enhance his overall wellbeing and happiness. These include opportunities for socialisation and interaction, and for adult learning, including improving his understanding of his diabetes as well as healthy eating and physical activity. These could enhance his ability to self-care.

- Healthy eating – look at nutritional labelling for any snacks Derek buys for himself, balanced intake (Eatwell Plate), portion size and speed of eating. Dietary changes should be kept simple.
- Physical activity – introducing increased activity gradually and incrementally, beginning with interrupting continuous sedentary behaviour.

Consideration of health promotion programmes that combine healthy eating and physical activity is also important. Having local knowledge of such resources in order to facilitate signposting is a key strategy.

Even those individuals who are have excellent control over their diabetes may experience periods of poor control, perhaps when they have a virus or are under stress, so all mental health professionals should be aware of how to manage acute situations should they arise.

When glycaemic control starts to be lost and blood glucose levels increase above 10 mmols/l (hyperglycaemia) symptoms start to appear: tiredness, increased thirst, going to the toilet more often to pass urine, sometimes blurred vision, feeling off colour. The mental health practitioner should check that all diabetic medication has been taken correctly and if possible test blood glucose to measure plasma glucose using a glucometer. Ensure that any extra eating of carbohydrate and/or sugary foods does not continue. Taking some appropriate exercise can often quite quickly reduce the blood glucose levels. Close monitoring should continue until the blood glucose level is within normal limits. Advice should be sought if glucose levels continue to rise or symptoms worsen. If the client experiences regular episodes of hyperglycaemia, this indicates poor glucose control and the mental health practitioner is advised to liaise with the client and the multidisciplinary team to explore strategies to enhance the client's glycaemic control.

People on combinations of diabetes medications can also experience hypoglycaemia, defined as plasma glucose <4 mmols/l. The person will have some of the following symptoms: sweating, trembling, anxiety, palpitations, headache, hunger, loss of concentration, deterioration in vision, disorientation and difficulty with speech, poor balance and feeling dizzy. As some of these symptoms are similar to the side-effects of psychiatric medication, they may not be obvious either to the individual or the mental health professional. This underlies the need for individuals to receive detailed and tailored education to facilitate their symptom recognition.

If possible, test blood glucose to measure plasma glucose using a glucometer. Even without access to this, treating the individual as though they are hypoglycaemic will not harm them, should this not be the case. The aim here is to raise the blood glucose levels to within normal limits and this can be achieved by using glucose tablets or dextrose tablets. If glucose is not available, use three teaspoons of sugar in a little water or milk; honey, jam, Lucozade or fruit juice can be used in the same way. In the event that the client is unconscious or unable to take oral diet and fluid, GlucoGel® (formerly known as Hypostop®) can be rubbed on their gums. Mental health professionals are advised to take glucose supplements with them should they accompany an individual diagnosed with diabetes to a place where food will not be readily available. The client should be encouraged to rest and, where possible, blood glucose monitoring should continue until it is within normal parameters. When the blood glucose level is 4–7 mmols/l, then hypoglycaemia is treated. If it remains low, repeat the process above. If there is more than 15 minutes to wait before the patient has a meal, give some starchy carbohydrate like a banana, a small sandwich, a couple of biscuits, crackers, or toast.

In some incidences individuals may intentionally cause themselves to become hypoglycaemic by overdosing on insulin, which can lead to a hypoglycaemic coma. In an attempt to prevent this, usually one month's worth of insulin is prescribed at a time and for people at higher risk of suicide smaller amounts may be prescribed at one time.

Clinical presentations of insulin overdose include coma, convulsions, transient hemiparesis and stroke syndrome, plus reduced consciousness and cognitive dysfunction which may cause accidents and injuries. Cardiac events may also be precipitated, e.g. arrhythmias, myocardial ischaemia and cardiac failure. If you suspect that a client may have intentionally overdosed on insulin, treat as a medical emergency and seek emergency medical support. Treatment will involve intravenous glucose therapy and glucagon if required.

Once recovered from the acute situation, it is very important that liaison between physical and mental health care providers is effective to ensure continuity of care and optimum outcomes for the individual client.

CONCLUSION

The prevalence of metabolic syndrome and diabetes among individuals with mental health problems necessitates mental health care providers having an understanding of these potentially devastating conditions. While health promotion, effective physical health assessment and care are central components of the mental health practitioner's role, ultimately the key to effective prevention and management of these conditions lies with the clients themselves. Clients need to maximise their physical wellbeing and enhance their self-management, and mental health practitioners are optimally placed to liaise with physical health care providers and support their clients in this endeavour.

USEFUL RESOURCES

At the time of writing in the UK we recommend the following resources:

Department of Health:
www.dh.gov.uk/en/Healthcare/Mentalhealth/MentalHealthStrategy/index.htm
www.dh.gov.uk/en/Publicationsandstatistics/Publications/PublicationsPolicyAndGuidance/
DH_123737

Diabetes UK:
www.diabetes.org.uk/Guide-to-diabetes/Food_and_recipes/The-Glycaemic-Index/
www.diabetes.org.uk/Guide-to-diabetes/Introduction-to-diabetes/What_is_diabetes/

National Institute for Health and Clinical Excellence:
http://guidance.nice.org.uk/CG34/QuickRefGuide/pdf/English
www.nice.org.uk/CG67
www.nice.org.uk/guidance/cg43

Government guidance:
https://nextstep.direct.gov.uk/Pages/Home.aspx
www.food.gov.uk/scotland/scotnut/eatwellplate/

Others:
/www.pharmanews.eu/lilly/359-diabetes-conversation-maptm-education-tools-celebrate-one-
year-anniversary
www.xperthealth.org.uk/

LIBRARY, UNIVERSITY OF CHESTER

4

CARDIOVASCULAR HEALTH IN MENTAL HEALTH PRACTICE

SIOBHAN TRANTER

Learning outcomes

By the end of this chapter you should be able to:

- Outline the structures and functions of the cardiovascular system
- Discuss the causes of cardiovascular diseases among individuals with mental health problems
- Explore the altered physiology of common cardiovascular conditions
- Consider how to assess cardiovascular health
- Explore interventions aimed at enhancing cardiac function for clients with mental illness

---

INTRODUCTION

Most readers will already be aware that cardiovascular disease (CVD) is of great concern to governments worldwide, not only for its cost to individual sufferers but also for the cost to the economy. CVD is now the main cause of morbidity in Europe (British Heart Foundation (BHF) 2008a) and in America it is estimated that more than 75 million people suffer from it. A worrying trend for the

American government is the rate at which CVD is growing in the 15–20 year-old population, suggesting that advances in health promotion are not having a significant effect.

Similarly advances in treatment are failing to have a substantial impact on the mortality rates of this disease, which continues to be the main cause of death in both Europe and the UK (BHF 2008a, 2008b). One in three deaths in the UK in 2006 was as a result of CVD, whereas in Europe almost half of all deaths have been attributed to CVD (BHF 2008a, 2008b).

CVD is an umbrella term for a variety of disorders including hypertension, coronary heart disease (CHD) and stroke. Of all the deaths from CVD in the UK, 48% were from CHD and 28% from stroke (BHF 2008b). In 2009, 32% of deaths in the UK were due to CVD. If these statistics are shocking when related to the general population, then they are more so when applied to individuals with mental health problems who are at least twice as likely to die from this disease. In the general population 8% of people are likely to die from CHD whereas the figure rises to 22% in people with schizophrenia (Disability Rights Commission 2006).

This chapter aims to provide mental health professionals with an understanding of normal and altered cardiovascular function to enable them to prevent CVD, assist in its early identification and provide quality care for clients with cardiovascular insufficiency.

CARDIOVASCULAR HEALTH IN INDIVIDUALS WITH MENTAL HEALTH PROBLEMS

Health outcomes and life expectancy of people with severe mental illness (SMI) are deteriorating and one of the main causes is cardiovascular disease (CVD) (Brown et al. 2000; Osby et al. 2000; Saha et al. 2007). People with schizophrenia have a mortality risk two to three times higher than the general population. In a study measuring the 25-year mortality of people with schizophrenia, Brown, Kim et al. (2010) found that there was a threefold increase in cardiovascular mortality comparative to the general population. Cardiovascular health is often compromised in SMI, with the prevalence of CHD estimated to be two to three times that of the general population (Filik et al. 2006). The *National Service Framework for Coronary Heart Disease* (Department of Health 2000) identifies people with SMI as a vulnerable group in need of particular attention. Moreover, there is a growing recognition of the part that depression may play in the development of CHD, yet Wulsin points out that 'we know so little about this apparently lethal exposure variable' (2000: 1132) .

The links between CVD and SMI are not confined to the UK. There is clear evidence that this problem exists in other countries. In the USA, Hennekens et al. (2005) identified that clients with schizophrenia are at twice the risk of developing CVD than the general population. In a Swedish study observing mortality trends, Osby et al. (2000) found that cardiovascular-related deaths in clients with schizophrenia had increased steadily in both women and men since 1976, while in New Zealand people with mental disorder were found to have a higher incidence of several chronic physical conditions, one of which was CVD (Scott et al. 2006). It has therefore been well documented and acknowledged that individuals with SMI worldwide are at a greater risk of CVD. Understanding CVD starts with an exploration of the anatomy and physiology of the cardiovascular system.

ANATOMY AND PHYSIOLOGY OF THE CARDIOVASCULAR SYSTEM

The role of the cardiovascular system is to transport oxygen, nutrients, heat and waste products around the body. The system consists of the heart and blood vessels. The heart is a dual pump. The right side pumps deoxygenated (without oxygen) blood to the lungs and the left side pumps oxygenated (with oxygen) blood around the rest of the body. The heart has four chambers: two ventricles and two atria and four valves which control blood flow. This can be seen in Figure 4.1. The aorta is the artery which exits the heart carrying oxygenated blood to the rest of the body. Immediately after it leaves the heart, coronary arteries branch off the aorta to supply oxygenated blood to the muscles of the heart itself.

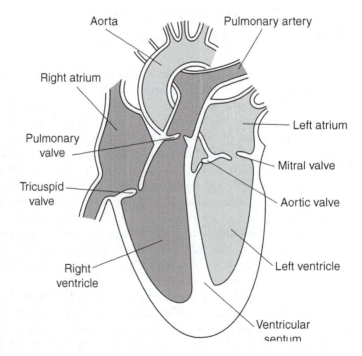

Figure 4.1 Heart

THE CONDUCTION PATHWAY

The pumping action of the heart is regulated by a series of electrical impulses which stimulate the chambers of the heart to contract and relax in sequence. This controls the effective flow of blood through the heart. The rate and depth of the contractions can be altered in response to changes in the body's demand for oxygenated blood, hence the elevation in pulse and blood pressure which are seen during exercise. The electrical impulses are controlled by a pacemaker called the Sino atrial node (SA node) which is situated in the wall of the right atrium. The SA node stimulates the impulses which can be recorded via an electrocardiogram (ECG), providing a non-invasive diagnostic tool that checks for disturbances to the rhythm of the heart (dysrhythmias).

The PQRST complex (shown in Figure 4.2) represents the normal rhythm following the initiation of an impulse by the SA node. As the impulse travels across the atria they contract, forcing the blood down into the ventricles (this is represented by the P wave). The larger QRS complex shows the atria relaxing while the bigger ventricles contract and push the blood up and out of the heart to the lungs (right side) and the rest of the body (left side). Lastly, the ST segment reflects the relaxation of the ventricles as they prepare for the next impulse.

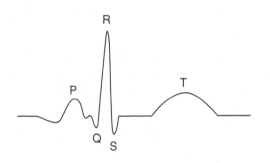

Figure 4.2 PQRST

BLOOD VESSELS

There are three types of blood vessels: arteries, veins and capillaries. Arteries carry oxygenated (except for the pulmonary artery) blood away from the heart to the limbs and organs of the body. They have thick muscular walls to allow the flow of blood at high speed and pressure. When the artery is near the surface of the body, the ripple of pressure can be felt as a 'pulse'. Arteries become smaller and smaller as they branch off into the tissues of the body and become arterioles before eventually becoming capillaries.

Capillaries are the smallest vessels of the body and are only one cell thick, which allows the perfusion of substances into and from the surrounding cells. The capillaries supply oxygen and nutrients to the cells and absorb waste products and carbon dioxide from them. They then join up and widen to become venules and then widen yet further to become veins, which return to the right side of the heart and on to the lungs for reoxygenation. Veins have thinner walls and larger diameters than arteries and are lined with valves which help the blood flow against gravity.

Veins and arteries can dilate (vasodilation) and contract (vasoconstriction) to direct the flow of blood. For example, the vessels in the skin dilate in hot temperatures to aid heat loss. This function is vital to the health of the cardiovascular system as it plays an important part in regulating the pressure of the blood within the vessels (blood pressure). The cardiovascular system is complex and multifaceted and deficits within any part of the system can have a detrimental effect on overall health.

ALTERED PHYSIOLOGY OF THE CARDIOVASCULAR SYSTEM

CVDs are a class of diseases that affect the cardiovascular system. They all share similar causes, mechanisms and treatments. In essence, the cardiovascular system is compromised when the flow of blood through the heart and/or vessels is obstructed or decreased, denying the body's tissues sufficient oxygen and nutrients. Such obstruction is commonly caused by degenerative changes in the health of the cardiovascular structures; the walls of the vessels thicken and lose elasticity both as part of the aging process and also as a result of smoking and excess salt in the diet. The lumen of the vessels is also reduced by the build-up of waste products such as cholesterol (fatty substance found in blood), atherosclerosis, which occurs when fat, cholesterol and other substances build up in the walls of arteries, and form hard structures called plaques and blood clots.

In recent years the term 'metabolic syndrome' has been used to describe a group of risk factors which occur together and increase the risk of CVD and type 2 diabetes (T2DM). While the potential to develop T2DM has been discussed in Chapter 3, the progression to CVD will be explored further here.

As noted in the previous chapter, Carmena (2003) estimates that the prevalence of metabolic syndrome in the general population varies between 11% and 53% across different countries, with increased levels found in western societies and among older age groups. The American Heart Association (www.heart.org) and the National Heart, Lung and Blood Institute (www.nhlbi.nih.gov) define metabolic syndrome as 'a constellation of interrelated underlying metabolic risk factors that appear to directly cause the development of atherosclerotic cardiovascular disease'. Simple clinical criteria to diagnose metabolic syndrome are set out in Table 4.1. Three or more of these constitute metabolic syndrome.

Individuals with metabolic syndrome commonly show an abnormal lipid profile (low good cholesterol, high bad cholesterol and high fat in the blood)

Table 4.1 Common physical findings associated with metabolic syndrome

Waist size	>40 inches in men or >35 inches in women
Raised triglycerides (fat in the blood)	>/= 150 mg/dl
Low levels of high density lipid (HCL) cholesterol (good cholesterol)	<40 mg/dl in men or <50 mg/dl in women
Raised blood pressure	>/= 130/85 mmHg
Raised fasting plasma glucose	>/= 100 mg/dl

Adapted from Grundy et al. (2005)

Source: Grundy, S. M. (2005) 'Metabolic syndrome scientific statement by the American Heart Association and the National Heart, Lung and Blood Institute', *Arterioscl Thromb Vas Biol*, 24: 2243–44.

which results in the accumulation of fatty materials in the vessels. Cholesterol, fats and other substances build up in the walls of the arteries and trigger an inflammatory response, which causes arterial hardening and the development of atherosclerotic plaques or atheroma. Over time, these plaques can block the arteries and cause symptoms and problems throughout the body. Atherosclerosis is also associated with the formation of a blood clot within vessels. In both cases the blood flow, and therefore the transportation of oxygen in the body, is compromised.

HYPERTENSION

Hypertension, or high blood pressure, is a very common chronic medical condition in which the pressure of the blood is elevated. Classified as either primary (essential) hypertension or secondary hypertension, about 90–95% of cases have no obvious underlying medical cause (primary hypertension). The remaining 5–10% of cases (secondary hypertension) are caused by other conditions that affect the kidneys, arteries, heart or endocrine system. In either case, hypertension imposes an increased workload on the heart and can inflict multiple minor traumas to the walls of the vessels. This heightens the risk of CHD and stroke and makes hypertension the primary modifiable cause of the wider spectrum of CVDs.

CORONARY HEART DISEASE

Coronary heart disease (CHD) is a decrease or complete obstruction of blood flow through the coronary arteries which supply blood to the heart muscle. This results in cardiac ischemia (lack of blood) which is associated with the symptoms commonly known as 'angina'. The chest pain and shortness of breath which result from an angina attack usually resolve when the imbalance is rectified. However, if the imbalance is not rectified, then an acute myocardial infarction (MI) can occur. If the reduction in blood flow to the myocardium is impaired for more than 20 minutes the affected part of the muscle will die. The term for this is myocardial infarction (MI) or heart attack. This is a common condition that accounts for most CHD deaths.

The term 'acute coronary syndrome' is used to categorise these pathological processes together. It signifies a rupture of a coronary arteriosclerotic plaque (atherosclerosis) or thrombotic (blood clot) episode that results in the symptoms of ischemia or infarction. ECG changes and biochemical blood markers are used to differentiate between a diagnosis of angina and an MI, as the death of the myocardium (heart muscle) is reflected in the presence of cardiac enzymes in the bloodstream.

CEREBROVASCULAR ACCIDENTS

Cerebrovasular accidents (CVAs or stroke) are the result of a disturbance in the blood supply to the brain. The carotid arteries, which travel up the neck taking oxygenated blood to the brain, can become blocked in much the same way as the coronary arteries. Alternatively, a rupture in the cerebral vessels can cause a hemorrhagic (leakage of blood) CVA. In either event, a stroke is a medical emergency and can cause permanent neurological damage and even death. Transient ischemic attacks (TIAs) commonly act as a prelude to a CVA as they are a temporary episode of neurologic dysfunction caused by a short-term loss of blood flow to the brain.

CARDIAC ARRHYTHMIA

The heart's conducting system is vulnerable to dysfunction from disruption to the chemical balance of the blood, infections or systemic blood loss. Cardiac arrhythmias arise from irregular electrical activity in the heart which causes it to beat out of sequence and become ineffective. Common arrhythmias include atrial fibrillation (AF) in which the atria contract and relax at an elevated rate and in an irregular pattern, tiring the heart and leading to a potential cardiac arrest. QT prolongation is a ventricular arrhythmia, in which the impulse is delayed as it travels through the ventricles. This can cause fainting and can even progress to ventricular fibrillation (VF), in which the ventricles' efficiency is significantly compromised as they rapidly and randomly contract and relax, which can lead to death (Glassman and Bigger 2001).

CAUSES OF CARDIOVASCULAR DISEASE

Wheeler et al. (2010) suggest that the causes of cardiovascular problems in clients with SMI are both complex and *multifactorial*. There are many issues that contribute to the increased prevalence, including lifestyle factors, socio-economic circumstances and psychotropic medication. Often risk factors can be linked or one can directly or indirectly affect another, as this will become evident in the following discussion.

LIFESTYLE FACTORS

Obesity is defined as a Body Mass index (BMI) of 30 or higher. It is a condition that is also multifactorial and though, for ease of writing, it has been placed here under lifestyle factors, there are many reasons why a person may become obese. Interested readers are directed to Chapters 3 (metabolic syndrome) and 11 (promoting physical wellbeing) for further information on this. There is little doubt that obesity is a threat to health and in relation to CVD it is associated with hypertension and thus coronary heart disease. Allison et al. (2009) found that 42% of clients with schizophrenia had a BMI of above 27 compared to 27% of the general population. Similarly, McEvoy et al. (2005) suggest that abdominal obesity affected 35% of men and 76% of women with SMI compared to 25% and 57% respectively in a comparison group. Clients with schizophrenia may experience obesity for many reasons, including inactive lifestyle, poor diet, the effect of medication or a lack of physical exercise.

Lack of physical exercise among mental health clients may be caused by several factors. Medication, for instance, may have sedative side-effects or clients may face decreased motivation levels or lack the confidence to participate in exercise. This problem may be compounded by limited finances, thereby rendering exercise an expense that cannot be accommodated. Financial implications could also affect dietary choices.

Furthermore, low income and reduced living conditions can lead to clients relying on convenience foods. McCreadie (2003) found that on average clients with mental health problems were eating 17 portions of fruit and vegetables per week compared to the suggested 35 (Department of Health 2004a). The same author also found that individuals with schizophrenia were consuming less fibre and vitamins than the general population. Another element of poor diet in people with schizophrenia was reported by Stokes (2003), who found a tendency towards increased sugar consumption.

Smoking

In a longitudinal study exploring the mortality of individuals with schizophrenia, Brown, Leith et al. (2010) identified that 73% of the cohort in the study were cigarette smokers. This figure compares to 21% of the adult general population in England who reported smoking in 2008 (National Health Service Information Centre 2010). Several older studies (McNeil 2001; De Leon et al. 2002) identify a similar increase in smoking in clients with mental health problems. There is also evidence to suggest that the genetic variant alpha7 nicotine receptor linked with schizophrenia could reinforce smoking behaviour.

Cigarette smoking is a major risk factor for angina and myocardial infarction. Tobacco smoke contains two cardiovascular toxins, namely nicotine and carbon monoxide. Nicotine increases cardiac workload by raising blood pressure and heart rate. It also reduces fibrinolysis and increases platelet aggregation which increases the likelihood of blood clots forming. Carbon monoxide reduces oxygen release in the tissues and causes epithelial dysfunction prompting atheroma (Jowett and Thompson 2007).

Alcohol consumption

There is a correlation between SMI and alcohol misuse. Individuals with SMI are three times as likely to be alcohol dependent as the general population (Weaver et al. 2003). In the UK, the recommended alcohol limits are <21 units for men and <14 for women. One unit of alcohol is equivalent to half-pint of beer, 25 ml spirits, and a 125 ml glass of wine, or 35 mls of spirits is one and a half units. Research suggests that as alcohol consumption increases (above three units per day) so does blood pressure, cardiac arrhythmias and sudden death (Lindsay and Gaw 2004). Although there is no evidence that confirms that alcohol consumption increases the risk of CVD, the Joint British Societies (2005) recommend between one and three units per day.

SOCIO-ECONOMIC CIRCUMSTANCES

Gender

There is evidence to suggest that CHD affects more men than women (BHF 2008b) yet this may not be the case where there is a co-morbidity of mental health problems. Goff et al. (2005) found in their study that when it came to mental illness it was actually women who were more at risk, and although they offer no insight into this finding, it is worth consideration as it goes against the common conception that CHD is a disease predominantly affecting men.

Informal and formal networks, relationships and customs within society provide a structure within which community and individual interactions take place. Being able to access and operate within this structure allows people to benefit from social capital which consequently can produce positive outcomes both economically and socially. An individual with CVD may, for example, benefit from accessing a self-help group which would involve a community interaction in a formal setting. Alternatively, they may prefer to access support from neighbours, which would be less formal and more individual, or even to access information and resources from a library or community centre, which is a growing part of current health care culture. However, McKenzie et al. (2002) suggest that for those in society who differ from the norm, exclusion is not uncommon and therefore social capital is reduced. This can be applied to people suffering from serious mental illness who often exist on the fringe of society.

Furthermore, there is some evidence that the way in which physical health care services are structured and delivered disadvantages those with a mental health problem. Factors such as clients encountering difficulties navigating health care systems, experiencing stigma or 'diagnostic overshadowing', coupled with problems in expressing their concerns regarding their physical health, may act to obstruct access to the services they require. A continuing theme of mental health policy is to reduce discrimination, social exclusion and inequalities in care, yet to date there is little evidence to suggest that this has proved effective.

PSYCHOTROPIC MEDICATION

Antipsychotics such as thioridazine, quetiapine or pimozide can cause cardiac arrhythmias (abnormal rhythms or rate of the heart). Some antidepressants and antipsychotic agents give rise to a prolonged QT interval of the ECG. This leads to an arrhythmia, ventricular tachycardia (rapid heartbeat that starts in the ventricles) and a condition called Torsade de Pointes (TdP), which can lead to sudden death (Witchel et al. 2003). Clients already at a high risk of cardiac complications should be closely monitored with ECG monitoring.

Clozapine, which is used to treat people with schizophrenia, has also been linked to myocarditis, which is the inflammation of the myocardium (the cardiac muscle). Symptoms are often non-specific and variable and can vary from fever to chest pain (Johnson and Rawlings-Anderson 2007). Most cases of clozapine-induced myocarditis occur within six weeks of commencement of the drug (Kilian et al. 1999). Initially, signs and symptoms will be non-specific flu-like, fatigue and fever and then progress to chest pain, shortness of breath and heart failure.

Finally, some antipsychotics are associated with dyslipidemia (high levels of lipids in the blood), which increases the risk of CVD. Other side-effects of some antipsychotics include increased appetite and weight gain (Dean et al. 2001; Wetterling 2001). Some drugs increase bad cholesterol and lower good cholesterol (Hennekens et al. 2005). All of these factors will increase the risk of CVD. Table 4.2 (overleaf) summarises the main conditions associated with coronary heart disease and lists the contributing factors for clients with serious mental illness.

Now take some time to consider Action Learning Point 4.1.

Action Learning Point 4.1

Identify the CVD risk factors for one of your clients. How might you go about assisting your client to minimise any of the modifiable risks?

THE ROLE OF THE MENTAL HEALTH PRACTITIONER

Appropriate awareness and knowledge of cardiovascular care is essential if mental health practitioners are to help address the physical health inequalities experienced by this group. Treatment approaches focus on physical health assessment (explored further in Chapter 2), health promotion (explored further in Chapter 11), and effective care of the client with cardiovascular insufficiency.

Table 4.2   Summary of conditions associated with CHD and contributing factors for people suffering from SMI

Disease	Contributing factors
Coronary heart disease	Obesity Smoking Lack of exercise Dyslipidaemia Gender Hereditary Depression Hypertension Diabetes Increased alcohol intake
Myocarditis	Antipsychotic: clozapine
Prolonged QT interval	Antipsychotic drugs
Hypertension	Obesity Dyslipidaemia Increased alcohol intake
Angina	Obesity Lack of exercise Hypertension Dyslipidaemia Smoking Hereditary
Myocardial infarction	Obesity Lack of exercise Hypertension Dyslipidaemia Smoking Hereditary Gender Depression

ASSESSING CARDIOVASCULAR FUNCTION

There is a growing assertion within mental health policy that individuals with mental health problems should have their physical health regularly assessed. While there is a lack of guidance regarding the specifics of such assessments, it is clear that a primary focus should be on cardiovascular disease risk management. Unfortunately, CVD often develops without the individual displaying any obvious signs and symptoms, and therefore can easily go unnoticed. However, routine physical health screening does offer a vital means of identifying individuals at risk of developing CVD and should combine subjective data, such as smoking and dietary habits, alcohol intake, exercise and family history, with objective measures, as follows (also see Table 4.3):

Table 4.3   Assessing cardiovascular function

Investigation/assessment	Normal limits
BMI	<25 kg/m^2
Waist circumference	Men <102 cm Women <90 cm (Asian men <90 cm, women <80cm)
Blood pressure	<140/90 mmHg
Cholesterol	Total cholesterol <4.0 mmol/l

Weight measurement

The most common way to measure weight is by recording the individual's BMI where weight is divided by height and then squared. This is a generally accepted classification that establishes levels that give an indication of the health risk posed by excess body fat. A BMI of >25 kg/m^2 is defined as overweight and >30kg/m^2 is considered obese. Table 4.4 shows the World Health Organization's BMI classification for adults.

Table 4.4   BMI scales

BMI range (kg/m^2)	Classification
<18.5	Underweight
18.5–24.9	Healthy weight
25–29.9	Overweight
30–39.9	Obese
> 40	Morbidly obese

Waist circumference is also recommended as a measure for visceral fat (fat around organs), which is thought to be more harmful than the fat deposited under the skin. Waist circumference is measured midway between the lower rib margin and the iliac crest (hip bone). If the measurement is above 102 cm in men and 88 cm in women, central obesity is present. However, in Asian populations lower values are more appropriate (Men >90 cm and women >80 cm). Individuals with SMI should have both their BMI and waist measurements checked regularly.

Blood pressure measurement

The National Institute for Health and Clinical Excellence (NICE) (2006d) has produced guidelines for the assessment and management of adults with hypertension. It defines hypertension as persistent raised blood pressure above 140/90 mmHg.

Hypertension is a major, modifiable contributing factor to cardiovascular disease (CVD). The aim of a cardiovascular risk assessment is to assess people's risk before CVD develops and monitoring for persistently raised blood pressure (BP) is one way to do this. BP should be measured on at least three occasions and be above the limit on all three occasions before a diagnosis is made. The NICE guidelines (2006d) offer the following clear and explicit advice regarding the way in which blood pressure measurement should be conducted:

1   Standardise the environment:

    • relaxed environment with the client seated
    • arm out stretched and supported, in line with mid sternum.

2   Wrap the cuff with correct size bladder around upper arm and connect to manometer.
3   Palpate brachial pulse in antecubital fossa (triangular cavity of the inside of the elbow) of that arm.
4   Inflate cuff to 20 mmHg above the point when brachial pulse stops.
5   Deflate the cuff and note the pressure when the pulse re appears: systolic pressure.
6   Re-inflate the cuff to 20 mmHg above where the pulse disappears.
7   Apply the stethoscope directly on to the skin at the brachial artery.
8   Slowly deflate the cuff and listen for Korotkoff sounds.

    • Phase 1: faint clear tapping sounds gradually increasing and lasting for at least two consecutive beats: note systolic pressure
    • Phase 2: sounds often soften and swish
    • Auscultatory gap: in some patients sound may disappear
    • Phase 3: return of sharper, crisper sounds
    • Phase 4: distinct muffing sounds becoming soft and blowing
    • Phase 5: the point where all sounds disappear completely: note the diastolic pressure

9   Deflate the cuff completely and remove from the arm.
10 Record reading. (NICE 2006d)

If the client is hypertensive on the first occasion, then the practitioner should provide lifestyle advice on ways to reduce blood pressure and schedule a further reading. If the individual's BP is less than 140/90 mmHg on further assessment, then their BP can be recorded annually. If, on the other hand, the client remains hypertensive on three separate occasions, medical advice should be sought. A formal CVD risk assessment will then be carried out with a view to commencement of drug therapy and further investigations.

Cholesterol levels

Non-fasting blood samples can be taken to measure cholesterol levels which provide a reliable calculation of CVD risk. The target level is <4.0 mmol/l of total cholesterol. The Joint British Societies (JBS) (2005) advice is that all adults over the age of 40 should have their total cholesterol measured as part of CVD assessment at regular intervals. For people with CVD or who are a high risk of developing CVD, blood lipid levels should also be monitored annually. Table 4.3 above provides the normal parameters of these investigations for an adult.

In the event that the assessment process identifies a client at high risk of developing CVD, health promotion and education activities should be initiated with the aim of lowering the risk where possible.

The JBS have produced a Cardiovascular Risk chart, available in the *British National Formulary* (British Formulary Committee 2010), which uses the data discussed in this chapter as a means of estimating the likelihood that an individual will develop CVD within the proceeding 10 years. The results determine a risk at <10%, 10–12% or >20% and can act as a guide to aid clinical decision-making regarding the intensity of any intervention.

Mental health professionals may also benefit from having an awareness of the discrete indicators of cardiovascular insufficiency which may be evident in their clients. These include signs of poor circulation such as discoloration of the nail beds, shortness of breath, peripheral oedema (swollen ankles or limbs) or general fatigue. It is also imperative that any episodes of numbness or weakness on one side of the body, dizziness, confusion or difficulty speaking and vision problems are thoroughly investigated as the client may be suffering from transient ischaemic attacks (TIAs).

FAST is a mnemonic which formed the basis of a public safety campaign in the UK aimed at detecting and enhancing responsiveness to the needs of potential **stroke** victims. Each letter of the mnemonic should prompt a series of questions which detects the classic signs of a stroke, as follows:

- **Facial** weakness – can the person smile? Has their mouth or eye drooped?
- **Arm** weakness – can the person raise both arms?
- **Speech** problems – can the person speak clearly and understand what you say?
- **Time** to call for help – if the person shows any one of these signs, call an ambulance.

Now spend some time reflecting on the assessment processes you utilise in your practice by completing Action Learning Point 4.2.

Action Learning Point 4.2

Reflect on your practice and

- Consider whether your clients receive the screening required to determine their CVD risk.
- Investigate the cardiovascular screening programmes available in your local area and whether they would meet the needs of your clients.
- Discuss with your team how formal cardiovascular screening can become a part of your assessment processes.

HEALTH PROMOTION

A Cochrane review by Tosh, Clifton and Bachner (2011) considered the effects of general physical health advice as a means of reducing mortality and morbidity and improving the quality of life of·those with a severe mental illness. They recommend that advice should not be given in a structured programme, but rather that programmes aimed at improving overall general wellbeing should be encouraged. Bradshaw et al. (2005) suggest that methodologically robust healthy-living interventions produced positive results in clients with schizophrenia and it would seem logical to suggest that the wider client groups experiencing SMI could also benefit from such interventions. However, Tosh and his team concluded that there was limited evidence that the provision of physical health care advice improved the physical health of clients with SMI. They advocate the need for more rigorous research in an attempt to provide an evidence base for this practice.

Weight loss can be facilitated by a combination of methods, including: diet modification, increased physical exercise and lifestyle modification. Diet modification means changing the type and quantity of food eaten. Eating less fat and sugar and eating more fruit and vegetables with an average calories intake of 1200–1600 kcal per day is often recommended. Some clients may benefit from referral to a dietician.

The cardiovascular benefits of regular physical exercise are apparent. However, it is recommended that, if physically able, 30 minutes of steady exercise five days a week is required to gain cardiac protection. Mental health practitioners will need to work with clients to establish realistic goals in relation to targets for both exercise and weight loss. Other factors, such as financial implications, motivation and self-esteem, may also have to be considered. Recommendations for mental health care providers' physical health care monitoring of clients with SMI include the Lifestyle targets outlined in Box 4.1.

Box 4.1   CVD Lifestyle Targets (Joint British Societies 2005)

- Do not smoke
- Maintain ideal body weight (BMI 20–25 and waist circumference <102 cms in men <88 cms in women)
- Keep dietary intake of fat <30% total energy intake
- Keep intake of saturated fats <10% of total fat intake
- Keep intake of cholesterol to <300 mg/day
- Increase intake of monounsaturated fats and decrease saturated fats
- Limit salt intake to <100 mmol/day (<2.4 g of sodium a day)
- Eat at least five portions of fruit and vegetables a day
- Limit alcohol intake to <21 units a week for men and <14 units for women
- Regular physical activity of at least 30 minutes per day, most days of the week.

CARE OF THE CLIENT WITH CARDIOVASCULAR INSUFFICIENCY

Despite the best endeavours of mental health professionals, it is inevitable that some individuals with mental health problems will go on to develop cardiovascular diseases. As such, the importance of effective liaison with the physical health care providers cannot be underestimated. Lifestyle modification aside, the priority in treating those with CVD is to lower the blood pressure and maximise the patency of the vessels, and the most effective means of doing this is via prescribed medications. Common medications include:

- Antihypertensives – There are many types of medication which lower blood pressure by different means. Among the most important and most widely used are diuretics which increase urination, thus reducing blood volume, angiotensin-converting-enzyme (ACE) inhibitors which dilate the vessels, calcium channel blockers which reduce cardiac muscle contraction, and beta blockers which reduce cardiac output.
- Blood thinning agents – Drugs such as warfarin, heparin and aspirin thin the blood, thus reducing the risk of blood clots forming in vessels and maximising the patency of narrowed vessels.
- Statins – These drugs inhibit cholesterol production in the liver. Research has found that they are most effective at treating cardiovascular disease (secondary prevention), but have questionable benefit in those without previous CVD but with elevated cholesterol levels.

For individuals with serious vascular obstructions surgical intervention may also be considered. Surgical procedures commonly include the use of grafts to bypass the area of obstruction or stents to hold the lumen of the vessel open.

Review your learning by considering the following case study.

Hilary

Hilary is a 58 year-old woman who has suffered from severe depression since the death of her husband 18 months ago. Six months after her bereavement Hilary attempted suicide by taking an overdose, which would have been successful had she not been found by a neighbour later that day. After a short period in hospital, Hilary was discharged home and she has been taking antidepressant medication since. She has also been receiving care from the community mental health team for the past year and is showing clear signs of recovery. However, during this period Hilary has lost interest in cooking or going out of the house and has gained a considerable amount of weight. She is also a heavy smoker and during a recent visit the mental health practitioner noticed that she gets breathless when she goes up the stairs. She is very pale, her hands are always cold to touch and she is complaining of feeling listless.

(Continued)

CASE STUDY

(Continued)

- What are Hilary's cardiovascular risk factors?
- What physical health assessments might you carry out?
- Are there any further assessments that you would advise Hilary to access?

Answer guide:

1   One of the most significant risk factors for Hilary is that she is a smoker. This, coupled with her depression and the related inactivity, renders Hilary at high risk of developing a cardiovascular disorder. Hilary's weight gain also poses a risk, particularly if it is centralised around her abdomen, while a lack of motivation to cook may have led Hilary to adopt unhealthy dietary habits, becoming reliant on foods that have a high fat and salt content.

2   Hilary would benefit from undergoing a physical health assessment and the mental health practitioner (MHP) could review her blood pressure, pulse, BMI, waist circumference and undertake urinalysis to identify the presence of glucose in her urine. In addition, the MHP could examine Hilary to identify any signs of poor circulation, considering her colour, pallor, and the presence of shortness of breath, discoloured nail beds or peripheral oedema. A detailed history would also be beneficial and should include Hilary's family and past medical history as well her lifestyle factors and barriers and motivators to change.

3   Hilary would benefit from attending her family doctor to undergo a more detailed review of her cardiovascular function. This may well include her cholesterol levels and possibly an ECG. Consideration should also be afforded to the possibility of Hilary undertaking a programme of smoking cessation and physical exercise. However, if Hilary is not willing to do this, then the MHP should utilise their skills in health promotion to encourage Hilary to make small incremental changes such as changing to a lower tar brand of cigarettes or undertaking gentle exercise to benefit her physical wellbeing.

CONCLUSION

CVD is the primary cause of the inequitable morbidity and mortality experienced by people with a mental health problem. As such, professionals working in the field of mental health are morally and professionally obliged to do what they can to reduce this. One way to do this is to utilise an understanding of the cardiovascular system and the CVDs that can arise and to monitor potential signs of ill-health. Another is to initiate health promotion strategies in a bid to enhance and support the client's physical wellbeing and this could all be enabled through the incorporation of physical health into existing assessment and treatment processes.

CVDs are progressive in nature and early detection of cardiovascular damage can prevent the development of disease. Mental health practitioners, through their enhanced relationships with clients, are in an excellent position to participate in this early detection and therefore to prevent the progression of further ill-health. In doing so, not only will they be assisting their clients to holistic health, but they will be impacting on the rate in which CVDs are currently cutting so many lives short.

USEFUL RESOURCES

At the time of writing in the UK we recommend the following resources:

British Heart Foundation – www.bhf.org.uk
European Heart Health Charter – www.heartcharter.org
World Heart Federation – www.world-heart-federation.org
American Heart Association – www.heart.org
National Heart, Lung and Blood Institute – www.nhlbi.nih.gov

5

RESPIRATORY HEALTH IN MENTAL HEALTH PRACTICE

EVE COLLINS

Learning outcomes

By the end of this chapter you should be able to:

- Outline the structures of the respiratory system and their functions
- Identify the causes of respiratory disease among individuals with mental health problems
- Discuss the altered physiology of common respiratory conditions
- Consider how to assess respiratory health
- Demonstrate an understanding of the effects of smoking on the respiratory system
- Discuss the ways in which the respiratory function of individuals with mental health problems can be enhanced

---

INTRODUCTION

Respiratory diseases represent a major cause of death and disability across the globe. The World Health Organization (2002a) estimates that 17.4% of all deaths and 13.3% of all disability adjusted life years (DALYs) are attributable to respiratory illnesses such as asthma, chronic obstructive pulmonary disorder (COPD) and pneumonia. Respiratory disorders are often progressive and gradually make daily activities more difficult to perform, affecting physical, social and mental wellbeing. People with a serious mental illness are significantly more likely to suffer from these physically debilitating and life-limiting respiratory disorders than the general population. This chapter aims to provide mental health professionals with an understanding of normal and altered respiratory function to enable them to identify current and pre-empt future health problems among this client group. This may support mental health practitioners to initiate health-protective interventions with the aim of enhancing the quality and duration of life for individuals within this vulnerable group.

RESPIRATORY HEALTH IN INDIVIDUALS WITH MENTAL HEALTH PROBLEMS

International research evidence has established alarming statistics regarding the prevalence of respiratory disorders among individuals with a wide range of mental health conditions. One of the most comprehensive reviews of respiratory co-morbidity and mental illness saw Harris and Barraclough (1998) offer an insight into deaths from natural causes among people with severe mental illness (SMI). The findings indicate that people with SMI are at a significantly higher risk of dying from infections and/or respiratory disorders. Critics may note that the majority of this data emanates from an era of greater institutionalised mental health care, yet contemporary studies, conducted in the age of community care, substantiate the link between respiratory diseases and SMI (Brown, Kim, et al. 2010). Filik et al. (2006) used health survey data to compare the respiratory function of people with schizophrenia with that of the UK population. A total of 89.6% of clients were identified as having poor lung function compared with 47% of the general population. Similar work conducted by Sokal et al. (2004) suggests that the same can be said for individuals suffering from schizophrenia or bipolar disorder in America, who were found to have significantly elevated rates of chronic bronchitis and asthma.

Tuberculosis (TB) has received scarce attention among people with SMI to date. However, with risk factors including alcoholism, HIV, older age, substance abuse, homelessness, lack of health care, malnutrition, incarceration and residence in long-term care (Grose and Schub 2010), it is evident that individuals with mental health problems are a vulnerable group. Thus, mental health professionals should have an awareness of this communicable disease.

Attempts to establish the incidence of lung cancer in patients with severe mental illness have resulted in some controversial findings. Lichtermann et al. (2001) and Brown et al. (2000) found rates of lung cancer among individuals with SMI were twice that of the general population. Conversely, a meta-analysis by Catts et al. (2008) reported only a slightly increased risk of lung cancer among this client group, which is surprising given their elevated smoking patterns. Indeed, when adjusted for smoking and social deprivation, Osborn et al.'s (2007) data found that the previously elevated rate of respiratory neoplasms among the 50–75 year-old severely mentally ill was rendered statistically insignificant. This has fuelled speculation that there could be a protective genetic or disease-related effect reducing the risk of cancer for some individuals with mental health problems (see Chapter 6 for further details).

These statistics make a clear case to support those calling for mental health professionals to enhance their knowledge of physical health care. Yet a more persuasive driver is likely to be found in clinical practice, where the true meaning of the statistics can be seen reflected in mental health clients, many of whom may suffer from persistent coughs or find their everyday lives limited by their struggle to breathe.

ANATOMY AND PHYSIOLOGY OF THE RESPIRATORY SYSTEM

The primary function of the respiratory system is to oxygenate the blood. Carbon dioxide (CO_2) is produced as a by-product of oxygen (O_2) metabolism and is expelled via the respiratory system. The continuous and reliable functioning of the respiratory system is essential to human life and any disruption to the supply of oxygen, either by disease or environmental circumstances, is potentially life threatening. The levels of oxygen and carbon dioxide in the blood have a significant effect on its acidity and alkalinity, which are carefully controlled by the cardio-respiratory control centre located within the brainstem. Its role is to interpret signals from chemoreceptors and increase the respiratory rate in response to high CO_2 levels and decreases the rate should the CO_2 levels fall below the normal parameters (see Table 5.1). In this way the homeostasis of oxygen, carbon dioxide and respiration are maintained.

The respiratory system is divided into two sections: the upper respiratory tract and the lower respiratory tract.

Table 5.1   Arterial blood gases

Arterial blood gases	Normal parameters
Oxygen	11–13 Kpa or 80–100 mmHg
Carbon dioxide	4–6 Kpa or 35–45 mmHg
Ph	7.35–7.45

THE UPPER RESPIRATORY TRACT

Air is taken in via the upper respiratory tract which is composed of the mouth, nose, pharynx and larynx (see Figure 5.1). These structures are lined with mucus membranes which warm and humidify the inspired air, while hair-like projections called cilia line the nasal passages and act to filter out airborne particles.

THE LOWER RESPIRATORY TRACT

The lower respiratory tract is composed of the trachea, bronchi and lungs. The trachea and bronchi continue the work of the upper respiratory system in facilitating the conduction of air to the lungs while cilia constantly clean the airways by

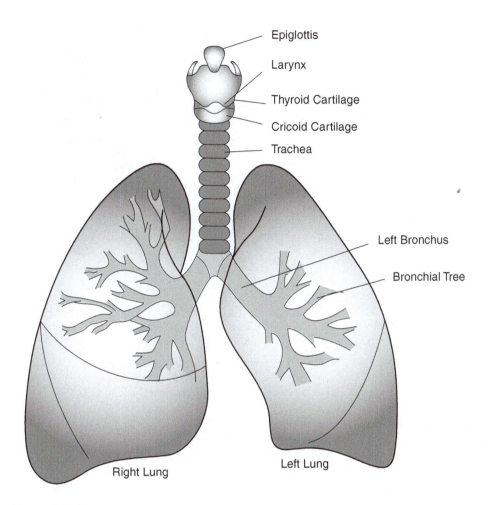

Figure 5.1 Lungs

carrying foreign particles up to be expectorated or swallowed. The left and right bronchi split off from the trachea before dividing into smaller bronchi as they enter each lobe of the lungs. Here they subdivide into smaller and smaller bronchi before finally branching into bronchioles. The air in the bronchioles is divided from the pulmonary circulation by a single layer of epithelial cells.

The lungs sit in the thoracic cavity encased by the thoracic cage. Pleural membranes separate the lungs from the rib cage and add lubrication which minimises friction when breathing. The right lung is divided into three lobes whereas the smaller left lung has two. Underneath the lungs is a concave layer of muscle called the diaphragm which divides the thorax from the abdomen. Each bronchiole feeds directly into a large number of tiny air sacs called alveoli which are swathed in a web of capillaries enabling gaseous exchange to take place (Figure 5.2).

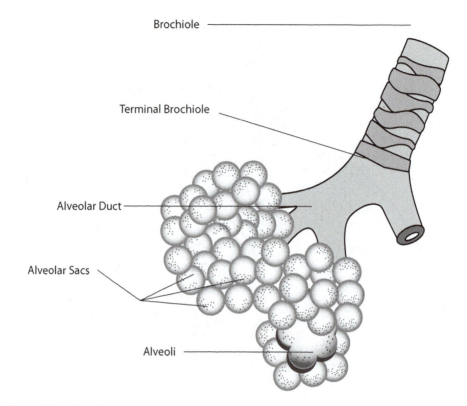

Brochiole

Terminal Brochiole

Alveolar Duct

Alveolar Sacs

Alveoli

Figure 5.2   Alveoli

RESPIRATION

Inflation and deflation of the lungs ensures a constant supply of air is delivered to the alveoli, enabling oxygen and carbon dioxide to be transferred into and out of the blood via gaseous exchange. This process of ventilation is an involuntary reflex. The respiratory muscles (intercostal muscles, diaphragm) work to achieve inspiration, which expends energy, while expiration is entirely passive. The muscles of the abdomen, shoulder and neck can be used to assist the respiratory process during difficult or deep breathing.

Ventilation is also influenced by a wide range of physiological variables such as the elasticity of the lungs, the degree of resistance in the respiratory tract and the effort required in distending the alveoli. Surfactant, an oily fluid, is secreted by cells in the alveoli and acts to lower surface tension, preventing them from collapsing or adhering during expiration. The lungs are never completely deflated, rather some air is always retained (residual volume), splinting the airways open and reducing the effort needed to expand them again. The cough reflex also plays a valuable role in responding to irritation or foreign particles by initiating a deep inspiration followed by fast, sudden, forced expiration, which expels any offending particles into the mouth under considerable pressure.

ALTERED PHYSIOLOGY OF THE RESPIRATORY SYSTEM

The respiratory tree is a delicate part of human physiology and by necessity the very air we breathe brings it into constant contact with the outside world. This presents frequent opportunities for the system to become damaged, thus impacting on its physiological function. Akin to many aspects of contemporary health care, respiratory medicine is awash with medical terminology and the reader is referred to the glossary should clarification be required.

Disorders of the respiratory system can be categorised into two groups: 'infectious' or 'obstructive', although they commonly co-occur.

INFECTIOUS CONDITIONS OF THE RESPIRATORY SYSTEM

The warm moist conditions in the respiratory tract make it an ideal environment for viruses and bacteria to thrive and as a result respiratory infections are one of the most common reasons people seek medical attention. The infection can be situated in the airways or in the lungs and may be of bacterial or viral origin.

Acute bronchitis is a very common, short-term and mild infection of the upper respiratory tract, usually caused by a virus, and often follows a cold or bout of flu. Such viral infections are usually self-limiting and resolve without medical attention within 7–10 days, although they can occasionally last for several weeks. Individuals experiencing acute bronchitis will commonly present with a cough, a mild fever, general lethargy, a wheeze and sometimes a burning or dull pain in the chest which is exacerbated when coughing or breathing deeply.

Pneumonia affects the lower respiratory tract and is a more serious type of respiratory infection, in which 'the alveoli become filled up with secretions and mucus, limiting gaseous exchange and, depending on the severity, resulting in hypoxia' (Watson 2008: 28). In the majority of cases, pneumonia is caused by bacteria, although in some cases it can be viral. The severity of pneumonia can vary widely, depending on the size and the area of the lung affected and the general physical health of the individual. Pneumonia can be differentiated from acute bronchitis by the presence of a high fever, shortness of breath and shaking chills.

Tuberculosis (TB) is a bacterial infection caused by Mycobacterium tuberculosis and worldwide it is the leading cause of death from infectious diseases and the leading cause of death for individuals with HIV (Grose and Schub 2010). It is spread when one person inhales the bacterium in droplets coughed or sneezed into the air by someone with 'active TB'. Once inhaled, the immune system of 80% of people will successfully destroy the bacterium (National Institute for Health and Clinical Excellence 2011b). In the remaining 20% it lies dormant and is referred to as 'latent TB'. The person will not be unwell or infectious, however it may later develop into 'active TB', destroying tissue and creating nodular lesions which fill with fluid. TB primarily affects the respiratory system but can also spread to the musculoskeletal, gastro-intestinal, cardiovascular, neurological and genitourinary systems. People with active TB may present with chest pain, blood in their sputum, fever, persistent cough (longer than three weeks), weight loss, loss of appetite, night sweats and shortness of breath, and should be referred to their family doctor. TB can be detected by a simple skin prick test and both latent and active TB are treatable with a prolonged period of antibiotic therapy.

OBSTRUCTIVE CONDITIONS OF THE RESPIRATORY SYSTEM

Obstructive diseases result from the airway narrowing or a lack of elasticity in the lungs which obstruct the airflow in and/or out of the lungs. The causes of obstructive diseases are multifactorial and arise from a complex interaction of genetic and environmental factors.

Asthma is among the most common. Sears (2008: 12) defines asthma as 'variable airflow obstruction'. In essence, asthma is a hypersensitivity of the lungs which is characterised by chronic airway inflammation with acute episodes commonly referred to as 'asthma attacks'. Acute episodes occur when a person with asthma comes into contact with a trigger (dust mite, pollen, etc.), which cause the muscles around the walls of the airways to tighten so that the airways become narrower and the mucosal membrane lining the airways becomes inflamed and starts to swell. Excess mucus is produced and then builds up, narrowing the airways further. The symptomology of asthma includes coughing, wheezing, shortness of breath and tightness in the chest (Asthma UK 2011), although the level of severity varies widely with some asthmatics suffering these symptoms all of the time while others have very occasional episodes of varying severity.

Chronic Obstructive Pulmonary Disease (COPD) is characterised by airflow obstruction that is usually progressive, not fully reversible and does not change markedly over several months (NICE 2010a). This umbrella term is used in relation to a range of conditions which are usually caused by smoking, resulting in permanent airway obstruction, including **chronic bronchitis** and **emphysema**. Most people with COPD have both. Bronchitis is a disorder in which there is excess mucus secretion in the lungs causing a permanent cough. Emphysema is damage to the alveoli of the lungs resulting in a loss of elasticity such that they collapse and stick together on expiration, making inspiration difficult. The process of inhaling air and prizing the alveoli apart expends additional oxygen from the already depleted circulating levels. The body has an automatic response to this which can be seen in clients with COPD who purse their lips on expiration which helps to splint some air in the lungs and prevents alveolar collapse. The symptoms of COPD include a productive cough, breathlessness and a wheeze, recurrent chest infections and other more vague symptoms such as weight loss, tiredness and ankle swelling. There is no cure for COPD and the treatment is aimed at maximising the client's quality of life and slowing down the progress of the disease.

CAUSES OF RESPIRATORY DYSFUNCTION

If you were to ask people working in the field of mental health why they think their clients suffer from disproportionately high rates of respiratory morbidity, most would attribute it to elevated rates of smoking. Indeed, there is substantial evidence to justify this assertion and it is no surprise that in an era in which we are becoming increasingly aware of our personal responsibility for our health, it is the lifestyle choices made by individuals with mental health problems which have attracted the most attention. While some conditions, for instance asthma, have familial links, it is lifestyle factors such as smoking, drug and alcohol use which have been shown to have a significant detrimental effect on respiratory function.

SMOKING

There are numerous epidemiological studies which have established international prevalence rates of smoking among people with SMI, up to three times higher than that of the general population (Brown et al. 1999; Kelly and McCreadie 2000; De Leon et al. 2002). Further, Kelly and McCreadie (2000) point out that not only are those with a mental illness more likely to smoke, but they are also more likely to be very heavy smokers.

We are all aware that cigarette smoke is detrimental to health, even though the mechanism of damage to the lungs and respiratory tract is less well understood. The toxic particles of tobacco smoke cause harm throughout the respiratory tree. One of the effects of cigarette smoke is to damage the cilia lining the upper respiratory tract and inhibit their ability to cleanse the airway surface. This reduction in mucocilary clearance is compounded by an enlargement of the mucus-producing cells which causes them to secrete excessive mucus. The body attempts to rectify this problem by coughing more frequently to clear the mucus, hence the resultant 'smokers' cough'. Both the smoke particles and the heat of inhaled cigarette fumes also damage the mucosa of the respiratory tract, causing inflammation and thickening, which constricts the airways and can also reduce a smoker's vocal pitch. Further, the delicate alveoli are also impaired by the build-up of toxins in the lungs which impedes gaseous exchange and causes shortness of breath. The presence of toxins in inhaled cigarette smoke also causes the body to produce additional white blood cells (WBC) which are believed to contribute to vascular injury and the development of atherosclerosis.

Stopping smoking will halt any damage to the respiratory system. However, the impairment to the alveoli cannot be fully reversed. On a more positive note, the inflammation of the airways will be reduced, cilia will regrow, mucus production will decline and the white cell count will return to within normal parameters. During the initial period after stopping smoking many people will experience an increase in coughing due to the mucosal irritation caused by the regrowth of cilia. A failure to anticipate this can result in the demotivation of potential quitters who may perceive their physical health to have deteriorated since they stopped smoking.

The first step towards facilitating smoking cessation is to ascertain what motivates individuals to smoke and researchers have made sterling efforts to understand why smoking is so prominent among mental health clients. The addiction model is the most widely accepted understanding of why people smoke, yet it fails to explain the increased levels of smoking among people with severe mental illness (SMI). One theory which does attempt to consider this relates to the therapeutic value smoking provides. Nisell et al. (2009) contend that by increasing serum dopamine levels nicotine decreases some psychotic symptoms and increases the metabolism of psychiatric drugs, thus reducing the side-effects of their use. Some evidence also suggests that nicotine addiction and depression may share a genetic predisposition (Audrain-McGovern et al. 2004), while alternative hypotheses focus on the behavioural and psychosocial factors which make it so difficult for people with SMI to alter smoking behaviour (Lawn et al. 2002). To date, the reasons why people choose to smoke remain an area of controversy (McCloughen 2003), while the growing intolerance of smoking in western societies adds to the pressure to address this issue in mental health practice. This challenge cannot be underestimated, with many commentators suggesting that smoking has become ingrained in the very culture of mental health practice. In recent years many mental health professionals have been expected to adapt from working in an environment where accepted practice included the use of cigarettes as a form of currency to manage or reward clients' behaviour to being tasked with enforcing a smoking ban. It is little wonder, then, that many mental health professionals may question whether their clients want or are willing to stop smoking and may also feel woefully unprepared to have any real influence on this behaviour. Yet there is no denying that the most effective way to enhance individuals' respiratory health is to facilitate them to reduce or ideally cease smoking all together. Readers are referred to Chapter 11 for further information regarding smoking cessation. Now take some time to consider Action Learning Point 5.1.

Action Learning Point 5.1

If appropriate, ask your clients about their experience of trying to stop smoking;

- What factors motivated and/or demotivated them?
- What part could you play in reducing the demotivating and increasing the motivating factors?

LIFESTYLE FACTORS

It must also be acknowledged that the prevalence of respiratory diseases among those with a mental health problem cannot be explained by smoking alone. Filik et al. (2006) found that when allowing for lifestyle factors, including smoking, the disparity in respiratory function was not eliminated altogether. The British Thoracic Society (2006) state that in 44% of cases of respiratory death, social inequality is a contributing factor, which implies that the wider spectrum of health determinants may also be having a detrimental impact on the respiratory health and longevity of this client group. Respiratory function is known to be affected by socio-economic conditions such as social class, occupation and environmental pollution. Indeed Marmot (2010) refers to a 'social gradient of health' in which there is a positive correlation between social status and physical wellbeing. Given that it is widely acknowledged that a diagnosis of a mental illness negatively impacts on the individual's socio-economic circumstances, it is little wonder that they are at greater risk of respiratory disorders. However, to date, comparative studies have failed to compare the respiratory morbidity and mortality of those with a SMI with people from similar social backgrounds, so it is not clear to what extent poverty, poor housing and unemployment are causal factors, rather than the direct effects of mental illness.

PSYCHIATRIC MEDICATION

An additional risk to the respiratory health of people with a mental health problem can be found in psychiatric pharmacotherapy which exposes recipients to the possibility of a wide range of respiratory side-effects, including suppression of the cough reflex, nasal congestion and reduced white cell production. Thus the elevated risk of respiratory morbidity is highly complex and can be seen to emanate from the combined influence of genetics, harmful lifestyle choices, poor socio-economic circumstances, and prescribed and non-prescribed drug use. Now consider Action Learning Point 5.2.

Action Learning Point 5.2

Spend 10 minutes identifying all of the risk factors for one of your clients and consider whether you are able to help reduce any of these risks.

THE ROLE OF THE MENTAL HEALTH PRACTITIONER

Health professionals and the overwhelming majority of the general public recognise that the most effective means of enhancing respiratory function is to stop smoking. However, among mental health clients there may well be those who have failed to stop smoking, those who do not wish to give up, ex-smokers left with respiratory deficits and clients who do not and have not smoked but who have respiratory problems. It is therefore important to acknowledge that there is a great deal that mental health professionals can do to enhance this aspect of their clients' physical care that is far beyond influencing smoking practices.

Appropriate awareness and knowledge of respiratory care are a prerequisite of quality holistic care for people with mental health problems. Treatment approaches focus on physical health assessment (explored in Chapter 2) and effective care of the client with a respiratory insufficiency.

ASSESSING RESPIRATORY FUNCTION

Having an awareness of the signs and symptoms of deteriorating respiratory function will enable mental health practitioners to encourage their clients to seek medical attention at the earliest opportunity. This has the potential to enhance the client's management of chronic conditions, prevent acute episodes and possibly even death. In addition, it may act to improve the inter-professional relationships with physical health care providers, such as family doctors, practice nurses and respiratory nurse specialists, allowing for cross-fertilisation of knowledge and a more seamless approach to the care of this client group.

The purpose of a respiratory assessment is 'to ascertain the respiratory status of the patient and provide information relating to other systems such as the cardiovascular and neurological systems' (Hunter and Rawlings-Anderson 2008: 41).

It may be impracticable or inappropriate to conduct a detailed and intimate examination of a client. Therefore it is imperative that mental health professionals are alert to the overt cues which arise when people are experiencing deteriorating respiratory function. These include increased coughing and breathlessness, which may be evident when a client needs to stop on a walk they would usually be able to manage, or are unable to talk without stopping to catch their breath. The respiratory system is very adept at compensating for reduced pulmonary perfusion and makes changes to the way we breathe to enable the body to get sufficient oxygen into the blood. The individual may not even be aware of these changes, which may well signal the onset of acute respiratory distress or even respiratory failure. Should these signs become evident, the mental health professional can either refer the client to a physical health care provider for further assessment or carry out some or all of the steps of a structured respiratory assessment as a means of eliciting more detailed information.

A comprehensive respiratory assessment can contribute to the diagnosis and management of respiratory conditions, provides a valuable early indicator of problems and should be cognisant of a full medical and psychosocial history where possible. The following process offers a version of Hunter and Rawlings-Anderson's (2008) comprehensive respiratory assessment which has been adapted for mental health practice.

LOOK

Respiratory pattern
Observe the client's respirations for one minute and note the rate, depth, symmetry and pattern of breathing.

Increasing breathlessness
Although there is no accepted 'gold standard' for measuring breathlessness, tools such as the Breathlessness Scale, offered by the Medical Research Council (MRC) (see Table 5.2) in 1940, are recommended for assessing severity.

Respiratory effort
Indicators of increased respiratory effort include breathing through the mouth rather than the nose and nasal flaring or pursing the lips. The use of accessory muscles

Table 5.2 Medical Research Council Breathlessness Scale

Grade	Impact
1	Not troubled by breathlessness except on vigorous exertion.
2	Short of breath when hurrying or walking up inclines.
3	Walks slower than contemporaries because of breathlessness, or has to stop for breath when walking at own pace.
4	Stops for breath after walking about 100 metres or stops after a few minutes' walking on the level.
5	Too breathless to leave the house or breathless on dressing or undressing.

Source: MRC Breathlessness Scale adapted by Stenton, 'The MRC breathlessness scale', *Occupational Medicine*, 58(3): 226–7. By Permission of Oxford University Press.

to aid breathing is shown by movement and tension in the neck and upper chest muscles. In an attempt to minimise the work of breathing, the body may also amend its posture by drawing the shoulders up, bending over or holding the back very erect to enable other muscle groups to adopt some of the work of the respiratory muscles. Changes in breathing rate and rhythm or a lack of symmetry in the movements of the chest also warrant further investigation.

Cyanosis
Peripheral cyanosis is detected by observing the client's nail beds and peripheries (finger and toes) for signs of a bluish discolouration, while central cyanosis relates to a bluish tinge to the mouth and lips. The cause of peripheral cyanosis may be respiratory or cardiovascular.

Sputum
Note the volume, viscosity and colour of the client's sputum. Green sputum is an indicator of an infection whereas frothy white sputum is indicative of pulmonary oedema. Blood in the sputum may indicate TB, carcinoma or trauma to the airways, often caused by coughing. Thick viscous sputum may be difficult to expectorate, particularly if the individual is dehydrated.

LISTEN

Normal breathing sounds should be quiet and any noise associated with breathing should be noted as it may indicate a restriction related to the air entry or exit from the lungs.

Respiratory sounds
Ideally, a stethoscope should be used to perform an auditory examination of the chest. However, where this is impracticable it may be possible to hear clients' breathing without a stethoscope. In this event note the presence and nature (dry,

moist, etc.) of a cough. Whistling sounds should be recorded as a wheeze, which indicates airway obstruction, and it is useful to note whether the wheeze is heard on inspiration, expiration or both. Crackly sounds may also be audible; this popping sound is usually heard in inspiration and indicates pulmonary congestion.

History-taking

Any physical assessment is ideally contextualised with a detailed client history. Specific attention should be afforded to the client's detailed description of the symptom triggers for episodes of breathlessness, factors which relieve it, present and past smoking and drug habits, recent trauma, vaccination and the history and nature of any pain and medication. Clients who have suffered chest trauma, however mild (e.g. bruised ribs), should be encouraged to seek medical attention if they are experiencing pain on inspiration as the tendency to shallow breathe can lead to a secondary chest infection and pneumonia.

A comprehensive respiratory assessment would also include the use of chest palpation and percussion, which assist the clinician in identifying the presence of congestion in various areas of the chest. Blood gas analysis, pulse oximetry and peak flow readings are also useful adjuncts in the assessment process but require specialised training and, as such, are likely to fall outside the remit of many mental health practitioners. Any abnormalities that arise during the respiratory assessment should be investigated by the client's family doctor.

CARE OF THE CLIENT WITH RESPIRATORY INSUFFICIENCY

The importance of effective liaison with the physical health care providers cannot be underestimated when caring for clients with respiratory disorders. Professionals working in the field of mental health should also encourage their at-risk clients to be vaccinated against influenza and TB, and it would also be prudent to afford due consideration to their own need for vaccination.

Mental health professionals may also find themselves faced with clients exhibiting the symptoms of a chest infection and may be unsure when to seek medical attention. As differentiating between viral and a more serious bacterial chest infection is fundamental to ensuring that the appropriate plan of care is instigated, an understanding of the distinguishing features is beneficial. While most respiratory infections share common symptoms, such as a hacking cough and sore throat, the key difference between a viral and bacterial infection is that bacterial infections cause the sufferer to become systemically unwell and medical attention should be sought if the person is exhibiting any of the following symptoms:

- pyrexial (temperature >38 C)
- significantly unwell and unable to manage daily activities
- they are confused or disorientated
- they have a high resting pulse rate (compared to normal)
- they are breathless at rest, or become breathless more easily than they would normally expect with exertion

- they have a sharp pain in their chest when they breathe in (pleuritic pain)
- they cough up green or blood stained sputum
- they have a cough that lasts longer than three weeks
- they have a significant long-term health problem, such as diabetes, heart failure or any other long-term condition that causes breathlessness
- they have a wheeze.

A definitive diagnosis can be achieved by sending a sputum sample for culture and sensitivity, which would identify the presence of any infective organisms, and X-rays are also invaluable diagnostic tools as they offer a pictorial representation of the lungs. Bacterial infections and TB will require treatment with a course of antibiotic therapy.

Clients who are short of breath should also be advised to:

- drink plenty of fluids to maintain the viscosity of the mucus and be encouraged to expectorate to clear the secretions from the lungs.
- maintain an upright position, well supported by pillows or a chair, as this will help maximise lung volume and prevent aspiration when eating and drinking.
- adhere to prescribed medication regimes which are vital both in terms of preventing and treating any acute episodes of respiratory distress. In particular, attention should be afforded to ensure that clients prescribed inhaled medication utilise an effective inhaler technique. Web-based resources such as that offered by Asthma UK may prove valuable in assisting clients with this. However, this does mean that an effective inhaler technique is vital to the disease management. The research conducted by Adams et al. (2004) suggests that asthmatics with co-morbid psychiatric conditions have poorer control of their condition, and Schmitz et al. (2009) found that asthmatics with psychological distress had higher levels of functional disability. Indeed, Asthma UK (2011) list psychosis, depression, and other psychiatric illness or self-harm among the risk factors for fatal or near-fatal asthma attacks. Thus individuals with ineffective inhaler technique should be referred back to their family doctor, who may opt to utilise a spacer device which make inhalers easier to use or a nebuliser to deliver the medication in the form of a vapour.

For those with chronic respiratory conditions, effective self-management is crucial to maximising physical wellbeing and it is vital that mental health professionals consider how they might best facilitate their clients in this endeavour. Maintaining a diary may help your clients to identify triggers and detect patterns in the presence of symptoms related to particular activities, environments, times of the day or seasons, etc. This can then be used to avoid known triggers where possible and may enable them to detect the early signs of deterioration. Although McAllister (2004) cautions that avoidance is often difficult as most chronic asthmatics respond to multiple triggers such as dust mites, pollen, tobacco smoke, animal hair as well as stress and anxiety.

Clients should also be advised to engage in a process of self-monitoring by recording regular readings of their Peak Expiratory Flow (PEF). This provides an objective measure of the individual's maximum speed of expiration which is an indicator of airflow through the bronchi and thus the degree of obstruction in the airways. The best of three readings is recorded. Clients who engage in self-monitoring will be able to provide their physicians with valuable information with which to review their treatment and medication.

Pulmonary rehabilitation should also be given to individuals with chronic respiratory insufficiency and is aimed at maximising the individual's functional ability by teaching breathing and muscular exercises to enhance respiration and maintain muscle strength. Oxygen therapy may also be needed to increase the circulating oxygen levels in the client's blood. It is important to administer oxygen therapy to patients with COPD with care. The respiratory drive is normally largely initiated by an increase of carbon dioxide but in people with COPD the cardio-respiratory control centre adapts to prolonged exposure to high CO_2 levels and reverts to using low oxygen levels as the driver for respiration. This means that should a patient with COPD be given high levels of oxygen correcting their long-term hypoxia, the respiratory drive will be reduced, slowing and eventually ceasing respiration. Gooptu et al. (2006) recommend that all individuals with COPD should carry an Oxygen Alert card, which highlights the potential danger of over-oxygenation and specifies a target oxygen saturation level. It can be printed off from the British Thoracic Society website and completed in coordination with the general practitioner.

Web-based resources such as those offered by Asthma UK and lunguk.org may prove a valuable resource for suffers of chronic respiratory conditions. However, it is widely acknowledged that your clients' co-occurring mental health problems are likely to render self-management challenging. A study conducted by Chafetz et al. (2008) suggests that there may be some utility in devising health education and promotion interventions tailored towards enhancing the self-management skills of this client group. Multi-modal interventions combining aspects of physical health assessment, health education and promotion with lifestyle changes such as smoking cessation and exercise programmes are increasingly used to maximise the health of SMI clients. Mental health professionals are encouraged to use the extensive body of literature in this field to identify strategies and interventions which have the potential to meet the physical health needs of their particular client group. Now review your understanding of respiratory assessment and care process by considering the case study.

CASE STUDY

Jethro

Jethro is a 56 year-old man who lives in supported housing. He has a diagnosis of schizo-affective disorder co-morbid, over recent years, with COPD. For several months Jethro has been quite stable, mentally and physically, but for the last few days he has been complaining that he can't breathe. Since suffering from COPD Jethro has had a tendency towards believing that the air has been poisoned and the staff at the residential home have often been alerted to a deterioration in his mental state by reports of an inability to breathe. On this occasion, though, Jethro is clearly having difficulty catching his breath and his coughing has increased in frequency and intensity. He has on occasion coughed up mucus. His key worker even thinks that there may be a slight blue tinge to Jethro's lips and he suggests to the manager that it might be Jethro's physical health that is deteriorating, rather than his mental health.

Take some time to consider the following:

1   What do you think the key health concerns are in the above scenario and what might they indicate?
2   What physical symptoms might you look for to indicate that this is a physical health issue? And what assessments would you conduct to determine the current status of Jethro's respiratory health?
3   What plan of care is required to manage Jethro's shortness of breath?

Answer guidance:

1   The key concerns in Jethro's case are the possibility that he is either experiencing an acute exacerbation of his chronic respiratory condition or a rapid deterioration in his respiratory function.

2   Symptoms such as a productive cough, increased breathlessness, lethargy, pain, increased confusion and evidence of cyanosis would act as alarm triggers and may prompt a comprehensive respiratory assessment.

Such an assessment should include a visual analysis of Jethro's respiratory pattern and rate, together with any evidence of increased respiratory effort (e.g. use of accessory muscles). A full history from the care team and Jethro may also prove invaluable in identifying whether Jethro has become increasingly breathless or experienced any respiratory pain in recent days. If the MRC Breathlessness Scale (see Table 5.2) has been used previously, this may be used as a baseline, facilitating the identification of any deterioration. Listening to Jethro's respiratory sounds may also help determine if his chest is congested, while a recording of his temperature and pulse rate would indicate the presence of an infection. If possible, oxygen saturation levels could be monitored as this would provide an objective measure of Jethro's respiratory function and aid in the clinical decision-making process.

3   In the immediate term, Jethro should be encouraged to maintain an upright seated position to maximise his lung capacity, minimise his exertion, drink plenty of fluids to maintain the humidity of any secretions, adhere to this prescribed medication (including oxygen), conduct deep breathing exercises and expectorate excess secretions. In addition, Jethro should be referred to his physical health care providers for treatment of any acute exacerbation and/or review of the care of his chronic condition.

Medication also forms a central component of the treatment of many respiratory disorders and, as such, mental health professionals may benefit from an understanding of some of the commonly used drugs.

Corticosteroids (preventers) reduce airway inflammation, oedema and excess mucus secretion. Used prophylactically, inhaled steroids such as beclomethasone reduce the risk of exacerbation of asthma (British Formulary Committee 2011).

Bronchodilators (relievers) such as prednisolone may be used. Corticosteroids such as salbutamol may be used to relax the smooth muscles surrounding the airway, dilating the lumen which facilitates respiration. The dominant route of delivery for this medication is via inhalation as this delivers the drugs directly to the lungs, minimising the dose required.

Decongestants or **mucolytics** thin out the sputum, reducing its stickiness and tendency to clog up the airways.

Antibiotics are frequently required for clients with respiratory disorder who are prone to episodes of bacterial infection. In light of growing concerns regarding the proliferation of antibiotic-resistant bacteria, there is a widespread recognition that health care professionals and the public should be educated regarding their use. Mental health professionals may well find themselves in the unenviable position of trying to explain why a client has not been prescribed the medication they desired or advising a client on how to take their antibiotics correctly. An understanding of the mechanism of action may therefore be of benefit.

Unfortunately, widespread misconceptions surround this area of medicine. The most pervasive of these is the belief that antibiotics can be used to treat all infections. This is inaccurate because antibiotics have no effect on viruses and, as a result, prescribers are cautioned against such imprudent use. The regrettable effect of this misconception can be the client's perception that their physical health concerns have not been taken seriously. Effective communication to explain why antibiotics are not considered appropriate is key to addressing this problem.

Antibiotics work by gradually reducing the pool of bacteria present in the body and thus it is crucial that clients complete any prescribed course of antibiotics, even if they feel fully recovered. Failure to complete the course may mean that the residual bacteria continue to multiply and cause a resurgence of the original symptoms. Previous exposure to the antibiotics may also enable the bacteria to develop a resistance and, as a result, repeated courses of the same medication may prove ineffective.

Antibiotics may render the combined oral contraceptive pill less effective at preventing pregnancy. Therefore women taking oral contraceptives should use an extra method of contraception while on antibiotics and for seven days after finishing the course. Clients on antibiotics should also be advised against consuming alcohol as it can compound any digestive irritation which is a common side-effect of this treatment.

CONCLUSION

The prevalence of respiratory disease among the mentally ill makes respiratory assessment and care a vital facet of contemporary mental health practice. The high incidence of heavy smoking among people with mental health problems represents a huge public health challenge to practitioners, who are urged to make best use of their therapeutic and communication skills to support smoking cessation programmes. By being attuned to the early signs of respiratory insufficiency, mental health professionals will also be in a position to refer clients to the appropriate service providers at the earliest opportunity, which will optimise their future recovery. It is also imperative that mental and physical health professionals work collaboratively to ensure that the services offered to this group support and promote their wellbeing, thereby reducing the current health inequalities experienced by these vulnerable clients.

USEFUL RESOURCES

At the time of writing in the UK we recommend the following resources:

British Lung Foundation – www.lunguk.org
Asthma UK – www.asthma.org.uk
Global Alliance for TB drug development – www.tballiance.org
British Thoracic Society – www.brit-thoracic.org.uk

ONCOLOGY IN MENTAL HEALTH PRACTICE

MAUREEN DEACON

Learning outcomes

By the end of this chapter you should be able to:

- Understand the relationships between mental health problems and cancer
- Grasp some cancer 'basics', including what cancer is as a biological entity, its diagnosis and staging, and common types of treatment
- Carry out an investigation of local cancer health policy and guidance as a context for supporting an individual
- Discuss the role of the mental health practitioner using case examples to illustrate how cancer screening, diagnosis and treatment can be tailored in relation to the person's mental ill-health

INTRODUCTION

The relationships between mental health problems and cancer have been the focus of much clinical and scholarly interest. This can be approached from two different perspectives: people who develop mental health problems following a cancer diagnosis and people with mental health problems who develop cancer. There appears to have been much more scholarly work in relation to the former group of people. Specialist cancer treatment centres often include psycho-oncology services and they are likely to be involved with the care of both groups. It is widely acknowledged that cancer is strongly related to psychological suffering (Lo et al. 2008) and that many cancer patients develop a depressive disorder (Slovacek et al. 2009). Indeed, depression has been implicated in lower survival rates (Boyajian 2010). This chapter will concentrate on the relationships between adults with pre-morbid mental health problems and cancer, but will first set the scene with a brief discussion concerning cancer and the general population.

There are many types of cancer – over 200, all with their own specific disease and treatment profiles. Some types of cancer are much more common than others. For example, across the world lung and breast cancers are the most common and thyroid cancer the least. The lifetime risk of developing cancer is over one in three. It is primarily a disease associated with older age as about 75% of new cases are diagnosed in people aged 60 plus. Tobias and Hochhauser (2010) note that the life-time risk is likely to continue increasing in the developed world as our population ages and more and better screening programmes are implemented. The chances of surviving cancer have grown, but it still causes about 12% of deaths worldwide and is a leading cause of mortality in the West. However, this is very variable, ranging, for example, from 24% in North America to 4% in Africa. Survival rates can also vary across cancer type and gender. For example, in the UK 90% of women survive the skin cancer melanoma for five years compared to 78% of men, whereas only 6% of men and women survive lung cancer for the same period. These complex differences are of great relevance to the individual with cancer but may be challenging for the non-expert mental health practitioner to grasp in their entirety. Fortunately, excellent information is rapidly accessible via the internet (see recommended resources at the end of the chapter).

Cancer is a highly complex phenomenon and can be studied from many different perspectives and with varying degrees of depth. The knowledge available for each type of cancer and its treatment is in constant development. The aim here is to provide the mental health practitioner with enough knowledge to care effectively for the physical health of their client group in relation to this disease and to equip them to learn more where necessary in the context of caring for individuals.

INDIVIDUALS WITH MENTAL HEALTH PROBLEMS AND A CANCER DIAGNOSIS

Current knowledge about the demographic incidence of people with both mental health problems and cancer is quite limited and mixed. Given the huge complexities that both of these 'umbrella' terms represent, this is hardly surprising. For example, researchers may include different diagnostic groups under the term 'mental health/illness' and thus find different rates of cancer in these populations. Here the findings of two research groups are discussed: Howard et al. (2010), who reviewed literature regarding those with severe mental illness (defined as bipolar disorder and psychotic disorders) and cancer, and Kisely et al. (2008), who studied cancer incidence in Nova Scotia in people using both primary and secondary mental health services.

Howard et al. (2010) examined cancer incidence alongside risk factors. They found that the majority of studies noted that, on the whole, there was a lower incidence of cancer in people with severe mental illness. However, the incidence of lung cancer and breast cancer was higher than in the general population, the former being potentially associated with heavy smoking and the latter, among other things, with lower child birth rates. These findings have led researchers to investigate further questions, including whether schizophrenia has a protective genetic effect and whether the use of some anti-psychotic drugs might be associated with breast cancer. Despite the limited evidence about cancer incidence, Howard et al. (2010) discuss with more confidence the evidence concerning cancer mortality. This evidence shows that people with severe mental illness are more likely to die from cancer than the general population.

Kisely et al. (2008) used records to investigate cancer incidence and mortality in psychiatric patients in an area of Canada. They found that cancer mortality was higher in this group by 29% but that this could not be accounted for by a higher incidence of cancer. This higher mortality rate was worst for men. However, the incidence of some cancers seemed to be lower in this group and others are the same as for the general population. Because this research team included psychiatric patients being treated in primary care, they make reference to the association between depression and cancer survival. This relationship has been examined particularly in relation to breast cancer. There is some evidence that suffering from depression prior to having cancer impacts more negatively on survival rates than experiencing depression post-diagnosis. Kisely et al. (2008) note that such cases would have been included in their study.

While these two studies explored cancer incidence and mortality within different definitions of psychiatric patients, raising questions about many confounding variables and the limitations of the data available, they make the same important observations: that, with the exception of some types of cancer, cancer incidence is either lower than or similar to that in the general population, whereas death from cancer is higher. The researchers discuss why this might be the case and raise questions about possible inequalities of care. These have implications for mental health practice that are discussed below. Although the evidence is mixed, Howard et al. (2010) conclude that people with severe mental illness (SMI) receive less cancer screening procedures than the general population. Furthermore, they raise the matters of 'diagnostic overshadowing' – a term used to describe the failure of the practitioner to recognise a physical health complaint due to the person's diagnosis of a mental health condition (Jones et al. 2008) – and, in some national contexts, insurance limitations affecting access to health care where people have co-morbid conditions. Both Kisely et al. (2008) and Howard et al. (2010) are concerned that people with mental health problems may go for medical help later when the cancer is more advanced, leading to a poorer prognosis.

Having discussed relationships between those who have mental health problems and cancer, the chapter will briefly examine what cancer is as a biological entity, its diagnosis and staging and the main types of treatment used.

CANCER AS A BIOLOGICAL ENTITY

Healthy bodies contain trillions of cells which age and die in a normal, systematic process and they are replaced when they divide in a well-disciplined way. When a person develops cancer, cells begin to grow in a disorderly way and this interferes with their ability to carry out their work correctly. The uncontrolled cells form a tumour and, in time, they spread into neighbouring tissues. When these malignant cells split away from the primary tumour and begin to grow in another part of the body they are known as metastasis. However, not all cancers take the form of a distinct tumour mass. For example, bone marrow cancers – leukaemias – are caused by rapid growth of abnormal blood cells. These abnormal cellular processes are prompted by genetic damage, known as mutation and it is this damage that interferes with the normal, healthy process. There are multiple and interacting reasons why this genetic damage occurs, including inherited predisposition, exposure to carcinogens, immune system issues and lifestyle risks. It is thought that cancer becomes more common in old age because there is more opportunity for mutation to take place. Exposure to carcinogens, along with cell lifespan mistakes (e.g. a cell repair goes wrong) are known as sporadic mutations and these are understood to cause up to 95% of cancers as compared to inherited mutations (Almeida and Barry 2010).

CANCER DIAGNOSIS AND STAGING

The path to receiving a cancer diagnosis is usually initiated by the result of taking part in a screening programme, consulting a health care professional because of health concerns or following investigation of acute symptoms. It is accepted that the earlier the diagnosis takes place, the better the prognosis is likely to be, so initiating this diagnostic process in a timely way is clearly of critical importance.

Routine and regular self-examination to detect the presence of bodily changes is recommended in the case of some cancers – breast, testicular and skin (Almeida and Barry 2010), but the evidence for the effectiveness of these strategies is contradictory. However, they are more likely to be helpful than harmful. Formal cancer screening programmes vary across the world. In the UK, for example, there are screening programmes for breast, bowel and cervical cancers. In Japan, screening for gastric cancer is under review because this is where this disease is most common (Tobias and Hochhauser 2010).

Given the many types of cancer, its diagnosis can be a highly variable, uncertain and troubling experience. Diagnosis will take place subsequent to a series of investigations, many of which may be unpleasant and frightening, and this will be followed by a process known as staging. The purpose of staging is to inform treatment decisions. The basic staging system common to all solid tumours is the TNM system. It is based on the size of the tumour (T), the level of lymph node involvement (N) and disease spread (M). Each cancer will have additional indicators that are considered too. For example, in breast cancer, treatment decisions may be influenced by tests indicating hormone receptors, and in prostate cancer, prostate-specific antigen may be measured via a blood test. During treatment restaging is often repeated, allowing review of the current circumstances and continuing treatment needs.

TREATMENT TYPES

The particular treatment of an individual with cancer will be based on multiple factors including the cancer type and its stage. Treatment may be aimed at cure (most commonly taken to mean survival for five years post-diagnosis), the best possible management of what is likely to be a long-term condition, or at easing suffering when the prognosis is poor – palliation. Different treatment types may be used in different combinations or in isolation and clearly this has complex implications for the treatment experience. Radiation, chemotherapy and surgery are the most common types of treatment. Surgery and radiation are most frequently employed where a confined tumour has been identified, whereas chemotherapy has a systemic effect. Hormone treatment and biological therapies are also used. Cancer treatment can be lengthy and extremely arduous and may have very uncertain outcomes. Coping with this and working successfully through a process of psychological adjustment is demanding of the most mentally healthy.

Radiation therapy, used in the treatment of over half of people with cancer, directs x-rays at a tumour with the aim of eradicating it. Great accuracy is required in order to minimise any damage to the healthy tissue surrounding the tumour. Radiotherapy is given in 'fractions' – small daily doses over a period of several weeks and is usually managed on an out-patient basis. Some people will require hospital admission because of specific treatment ramifications. For example, radiotherapy to the neck area can make eating and drinking impossible, meaning that the patient has to be fed through a naso-gastric tube. It can also be delivered internally. Brachytherapy, as this is known, involves local implants of radio-active pellets. Radiotherapy can be a time-consuming process involving careful planning and preparation before the treatment starts. Experiencing radiation therapy can be distressing and demanding and it can have unpleasant side-effects (Faithfull 2008). These commonly include fatigue, skin reactions and enteritis, as well as reactions specific to the treatment site. Side-effects can add a long-term health burden too. For example, women receiving radiotherapy for gynaecological cancers may later develop bowel problems.

Surgical intervention is used for different purposes. It may be used as a prophylactic measure to prevent the occurrence of cancer in cases of genetic predisposition, for the purpose of diagnosis and staging via a biopsy, or for 'debulking'. Some solid tumours cannot be completely removed because of their location. Debulking can be used to remove some of it, either to relieve acute symptoms or to enhance the likely effectiveness of other treatments. Most optimistically, surgery can be aimed at removing a whole solid tumour and this procedure offers the best hope of cure (O'Connor 2008). This is sometimes referred to as definitive surgery. Like radiotherapy, the individual's experience of surgery will vary according to many complex factors but generally surgery may be frightening and debilitating, with both short-term and long-term effects.

While radiation therapy and surgery are aimed at specific local tissue sites, chemotherapy has a systemic effect on the whole body. It too can be used either curatively, as a method for controlling the disease, or for palliation. The purpose of cytotoxic drugs is to kill cancer cells but they disrupt normal cell processes too. However, normal cells are intrinsically more able to withstand and recover from chemotherapy (Dougherty and Bailey 2008). There is clearly a critical role for very fine-tuning in achieving a therapeutic effect from the drugs used, while avoiding too much damage to the healthy cells.

Generally, chemotherapy is administered intravenously and intermittently on an out-patient basis. It has immediate, short-term and long-term side-effects. Its unpleasant side-effects are notorious and largely associated with their impact on healthy cells that normally divide rapidly. These are cells in the gastrointestinal tract, the bone marrow, the hair follicles and the testes and ovaries. Damage to the mucosal lining of the gastrointestinal tract can cause appetite loss, mouth ulcers, strange taste changes, nausea, vomiting and diarrhoea or constipation. The bone marrow cells that produce platelets and red and white blood cells are destroyed by cytotoxic drugs and this can lead to dangerous, life-threatening side-effects. Low numbers of white blood cells (neutropenia) increases infection risk and depletion of red blood cells leads to anaemia, causing the experience of fatigue and breathlessness. Low numbers of platelets (thrombocytopenia) affect blood clotting and this can lead to bleeding and thrombosis. Total or partial hair loss may result from chemotherapy, beginning shortly after commencing treatment and being at its worst after 4–8 weeks. Some cytotoxic drugs and administration regimes are more likely to cause hair loss than others (Lemieux et al. 2008). Both men and women can find this side-effect very upsetting and socially exposing (Hilton et al. 2008). On the whole, hair will grow back but it may be different in texture and colour post-chemotherapy.

Chemotherapy can lead to infertility in men and women. Again, this will vary according to a number of factors, including the specific cytotoxic drugs used and the person's age at the point of treatment. Pre-menopausal women are likely to experience amenorrhoea and menopausal symptoms such as vaginal dryness and hot flushes during treatment. However, women should take care to avoid becoming pregnant as the drugs may have serious implications for the baby's health. Fatigue is a common and very debilitating side-effect of chemotherapy and worsens as the treatment progresses. There are many other side-effects. Dougherty and Bailey (2008) make the important point that patients' concerns about side-effects may be quite different from those expected by health care staff and this emphasises the need to be person-centred. When the chemotherapy regime has been completed, the recovery time is highly variable and this can be a very difficult time for individuals.

Hormone/endocrine therapy can be used for some uterine, breast and prostate cancers as they are hormone sensitive. The therapy is aimed at either preventing or reducing the cancer's growth. For example, a well-known hormone treatment for breast cancer is a drug called Tamoxifen. It is used for breast cancers that have oestrogen positive receptors and is normally prescribed for five years. Commonly, it can cause unpleasant sweats and hot flushes and, in pre-menopausal women, disruption to menstruation. The woman's periods may stop altogether.

Biological therapy, also known as immunotherapy is used less commonly than the treatments described above. It makes use of naturally occurring substances and defences within the body and there are several types, including gene therapy and vaccine therapy, which are largely in the early stages of development. Bridgewater and Gore (2008) argue that the use of these has been clinically disappointing thus far, but much has been learnt and research continues. Another type of biological therapy is the use of monoclonal antibodies. These attach to the surface of tumour cells making them more vulnerable to destruction by the immune system. A well-known type of monoclonal antibody is the drug known as 'Herceptin', used to treat a specific type of breast cancer.

In discussing some fundamental information about cancer and its diagnosis and treatment, the broad oncology context in which the individual with mental health problems and cancer will be cared for has been laid out. Clearly, the cancer experience will challenge the mental health of the most psychologically resilient, so it can be hypothesised that co-morbid mental health problems may lead to even greater vulnerability and suffering. A further broad context to consider is that of health policy and guidance. Familiarity with this will enable the mental health practitioner to understand their patients' entitlements to cancer services and, in turn, will allow them to be their supporters and advocates where necessary.

CANCER POLICY AND GUIDANCE

The World Health Organization (2002b) recommended that individual countries should develop national cancer strategies. Clearly, health policy and guidance will vary internationally and practitioners are likely to be well versed in how to find out this information. Two examples have been chosen to demonstrate its salience to good practice.

The New Zealand Cancer Control Strategy (Ministry of Health and the New Zealand Cancer Control Trust 2003) sets out to reduce the incidence and impact of cancer and to reduce the inequalities evident regarding morbidity and mortality, particularly within the Māori population. Cancer is the leading cause of death in New Zealand. The strategy has six goals, including better primary prevention and an improved quality of life for those with cancer. Each goal has an associated action plan and the next planned phase of the strategy is to assess progress and outcomes. While the strategy does not specifically address the needs of people with mental health problems, it widely acknowledges the need for effective and timely psychological care. Familiarity with this policy will enable the New Zealand mental health practitioner to support their patients in accessing the available oncology services and, where necessary, in promoting their service entitlement.

The UK Department of Health has published *Improving Outcomes: A Strategy for Cancer* (Department of Health 2011b). In common with the New Zealand strategy, it aims to improve outcomes across the cancer trajectory and emphasises the need to reduce inequalities. It refers to the National Inequality Cancer Initiative, a body charged with understanding and implementing change in areas of inequality, including for those with mental health problems. Furthermore, it notes an ongoing study into the relationship between bowel cancer and schizophrenia because, it states, an early study indicates that people with schizophrenia are 40% more likely to suffer from it. The provision of psychological care for all cancer patients is receiving growing attention in the UK. The *Psychological Support Measures* (National Cancer Peer Review–National Cancer Action Team 2010) clearly sets out a workforce strategy and implementation plan for its provision. As in the New Zealand case, these policy commitments offer UK mental health practitioners potential levers in facilitating and supporting good oncology care for their patients. Before moving on, take a look at Action Learning Point 6.1.

Action Learning Point 6.1

- Explore the national cancer policy for your country and consider how it can enable you to support your client group more effectively.
- Examine the national mental health policy for your country to see what it says about the physical care of people with mental health problems.
- Share your findings with a colleague and discuss any implications for your mental health practice.

THE ROLE OF THE MENTAL HEALTH PRACTITIONER

There appears to be quite limited scholarly evidence available to guide the mental health practitioner in their care of patients with cancer. Howard et al. (2010) note how a person's mental health problems and their treatment may complicate and compromise their cancer treatment and they recommend close liaison between psychiatrists, oncologists and psycho-oncologists. They refer to examples of good practice taken from clinical experience and in the absence of stronger evidence this is the strategy we follow below. Pal, Katheria and Hurria (2010) make a similar case for the care of older people with cancer, arguing for careful attention to health needs assessment and the subsequent tailoring of treatment and care.

Broadly, the role of the mental health practitioner is to support and facilitate the care of their clients across the cancer trajectory. In practice, this involves factoring in and responding, via tailored interventions, to the needs arising from the person's mental health problems in relation to their cancer. As discussed above, there are strong indications that people with mental health problems and cancer die earlier than those who do not have a mental health problem. Mental health practitioners potentially are in a strong position to address this disturbing health inequality. Of critical importance to effective intervention is the practitioner's mind-set, that is, does the mental health practitioner believe that this is a legitimate part of their work? And if they do, does the organisation they work in have the same perspective? Without this overall commitment it may be difficult to act in the person's best interests (Eldridge et al. 2011). Blythe and White (2012) note that role ambiguity among mental health nurses is an important matter and that such nurses often lack confidence in physical health care generally. However, growing concern about the physical health of people with mental health problems has placed this commitment into the mental health policy arena and practitioners can be guided by this. For example, in the UK, contemporary mental health policy (Department of Health 2011c) includes a clear objective concerning the need to improve the physical health of individuals with mental health problems, so clearly practitioners should regard this as part of their role. Taking this as a given, we move on to examine in detail how the individual's mental health can be considered by using mini case studies and drawing out practice principles.

CANCER SCREENING

Self-examination can be encouraged as part of an overall health promotion and self-care strategy and clients may require support in taking part in cancer screening programmes. Susan's case study illustrates how the mental health practitioner can provide such support.

Susan

Susan, aged 32 with bipolar disorder, has recently married and wants to have children. In preparation, she is keen to be as healthy as possible but has always refused to take part in cervical screening, fearing that it would just be too embarrassing and difficult. She lacks social confidence and finds it very hard to trust people. Susan has previously indicated that she was sexually abused as a child but has never felt 'ready' to talk about it. Gallo-Silver and Weiner (2006) discuss how these traumatic experiences can impede cancer diagnosis and treatment. Having received another invitation for screening, she decides to discuss it with her Community Mental Health Nurse. The nurse gently and respectfully encourages Susan to talk through the issues and they agree that trust is at the heart of the problem. However, they also agree that cervical screening is important and that if Susan becomes pregnant she will need to undergo vaginal examinations in the future too. The nurse suggests that they look at some information about cervical screening together to understand it better and to see if it is possible for Susan to have an appointment with the person doing the screening prior to the procedure itself, its

(Continued)

CASE STUDY

(Continued)

purpose being to discuss exactly what will happen and to get to know the clinician. This way Susan can be as prepared as possible having had her concerns heard with care and sensitivity, and the door left open to discuss her previous experiences if she so chooses.

Women with schizophrenia have high risk factors for breast cancer (Seeman 2011). 'Margaret' is one of these and her case study considers how best the mental health team can support her.

CASE STUDY

Margaret

Margaret is 54 years old and lives with her elderly father, who is her main carer. Diagnosed with schizophrenia as a young woman, she has been severely mentally ill for most of her life. She has a complex delusional system and is highly sensitive to new social situations where she can become paranoid and hostile. Margaret takes little exercise and eats an odd, highly restricted diet which she has steadfastly refused to discuss or change. While uncomplaining about any physical problems, she looks pale and seems to get out of breath easily. She has been called routinely for breast cancer screening and surprises her mental health social worker by stating that she intends to go, having seen a programme about breast cancer and screening on the television.

Her social worker has very mixed feelings about this: he is delighted that she is keen to take part and with what this says about Margaret's desire to care for herself, but he is concerned about how she will actually manage the screening event. He explains this to Margaret and sets out to discuss it with the multidisciplinary team. Following careful discussion, Margaret agrees that the social worker can arrange for her to have the first appointment of the day, to discuss her needs with the radiographer and to be accompanied by a female support worker she knows. The team have agreed that while this is a time-consuming and expensive intervention, it is both ethically correct and a good investment in terms of relapse prevention.

Take a look at Action Learning Point 6.2 and plan how to implement these.

Action Learning Point 6.2

- Critically consider your role in relation to supporting mentally ill people with cancer screening.
- Investigate the cancer screening programmes available where you live and how these relate to the needs of your client group.
- Discuss with your team how formal cancer screening can become a routine consideration during assessment and care planning.

FACILITATING PHYSICAL SYMPTOM INVESTIGATION

Consulting a health care professional because of health concerns requires both resources and skills. For example, making an appointment requires a level of personal organisation and motivation. Having got this far, people with mental health problems may face diagnostic overshadowing (Howard et al. 2010). It is easy to be simplistically critical of this process but with limited consultation time and complex patient presentations it may not be that surprising. Let us consider the case of 'Greg'.

CASE STUDY

Greg

Greg, aged 69, has suffered from disabling depression and anxiety for 25 years and has made several serious suicide attempts. He periodically binge drinks and is socially isolated, having become estranged from his family. Despite several attempts to stop smoking, he smokes 20 cigarettes per day. When acutely unwell he neglects himself and frequently complains of various aches and pains. During a routine out-patient appointment with a psychiatrist he complains that he has been to see his general practitioner about a painful cough and felt that he'd been sent away and 'told off' because of smoking. The psychiatrist, taking a careful history, discovers that Greg has had the cough for several weeks, has back pain when he coughs, has little appetite, has lost weight and has little energy, yet he does not seem to be depressed and anxious at present. With Greg's permission the psychiatrist contacts his general practitioner and sets out why he is concerned about his physical health, stressing how his presentation differs on this occasion and does not seem to be related to his mental health. Collaboratively, they agree that Greg needs further investigations, including a chest x-ray. By understanding the pattern of relationships between Greg's physical and mental health his psychiatrist is able to see that his current complaint falls outside that normal pattern and is therefore able to inform and facilitate his access to health care.

SUPPORTING THE PERSON THROUGH A CANCER DIAGNOSIS

Receiving a cancer diagnosis is overwhelmingly disturbing to the person and their family and friends. Wells (2008), noting what an intensely individual experience this is, argues that several matters can impact on these reactions, including the events leading up to the diagnosis, previous coping styles, personal perceptions of cancer and knowledge of the treatment likely to follow. Again, we also need to factor in the person's mental ill-health. Let us return to Greg's story, presenting alternative scenarios.

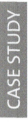

Scenario 1

Following the chest x-ray and further investigations, Greg is invited to an appointment with an oncologist. He has been encouraged to bring someone with him but does not. At the meeting he is told by the oncologist and a specialist nurse with great care and sensitivity that he has small cell lung cancer and that it has already spread to other parts of his body. This is common with this type of cancer (Almeida and Barry 2010). They continue to give him information about what treatment they think may help. During this Greg suddenly gets up and leaves saying: 'Well, that's it then. I deserve this'. On leaving the hospital, Greg commences a drinking binge and fails to attend any further appointments with either the oncologist or psychiatrist.

Scenario 2

Having facilitated Greg's physical health care, the psychiatrist asks the general practitioner to keep him informed and for Greg to come and see him again quickly. He refers him to the local community mental health team for extra support, where he is taken on by an assistant practitioner, who, in turn, attends the oncology appointment with him. She holds his hand and encourages him to listen, to ask questions and to clarify what will happen next. She takes him home, listening, supporting and comforting him, arranging to call back the following day to see how he is. The mental health team discuss his case and develop a care plan in collaboration with the oncology and community nursing teams. A few months later Greg dies peacefully in a local hospice.

Take some time out to work through Action Learning Point 6.3.

Action Learning Point 6.3

- Deliberate how diagnostic overshadowing might delay cancer diagnosis and treatment in your client group.
- Make notes concerning the actions you might take if you thought that diagnostic overshadowing was taking place.
- Imagine that a known client receives a cancer diagnosis and consider your role in relation to supporting them.

SUPPORTING THE PERSON THROUGH TREATMENT

The need to tailor care for the individual is not likely to be a one-off task, but more like a journey with lots of twists and turns, as in Ahmed's case.

Ahmed

Ahmed, aged 26, has been treated for a psychotic disorder for the last seven years. He has had several admissions to the local acute psychiatric ward, on occasions having been legally detained. He smokes cigarettes, has used illicit drugs and has volatile relationships with his family. Normally energetic and active, Ahmed has experienced persistent fatigue, flu-like symptoms and frequent infections. Supported by his family and mental health care coordinator (an occupational therapist called Gary) he has received a diagnosis of Acute Lymphoblastic Leukaemia (ALL). This is quite uncommon in his age group (Almeida and Barry 2010). His family are of the view that his current physical ill-health has facilitated the diagnostic process because Ahmed 'has been unusually cooperative and not his usual argumentative self'. The haematologist has explained that Ahmed's treatment will consist of several phases of chemotherapy and that this is his best chance of survival. Ahmed's response has been to agree to this plan, with the statement 'whatever'. Gary is aware that Ahmed's ability to concentrate on new information is quite limited and is concerned as to the degree that Ahmed has 'taken in' the demands and the effects of the treatment that he is facing. Gary is aware too that his own knowledge of ALL is extremely limited but understands that Ahmed will also need to continue on his anti-psychotic drug regime: being as mentally well as possible will enhance his health chances overall, as will a measure of social stability.

Gary organises a care planning meeting with Ahmed's mental health team, Ahmed and his family. In preparation, he finds out about ALL and locates some patient information for Ahmed and his family from the Cancer Research UK website. He discovers that anti-psychotic drugs can be dangerous in combination with cytotoxic drugs. During the meeting, a list of matters to be considered and acted upon are agreed – all in the spirit of supporting Ahmed through a difficult time and optimising his chances of recovery. These include, for example, a discussion between the medical staff regarding the safest drug treatments, the need for Gary to act as a communication 'switchboard' for everybody involved and to meet the oncology team to agree on a shared and documented package of support. After much discussion Ahmed agrees that Gary can inform the oncology team about his psychosis relapse signature, but only in his presence and that he is willing to *talk about* giving up smoking given that it will hinder his recovery. Gary commits himself to learning about the specific self-care that Ahmed will need to follow during chemotherapy, for example, taking his temperature regularly to check for infection. Despite effective collaboration and careful care planning, the mental health team and Ahmed's family remain concerned for the future. Ahmed's response to chemotherapy is uncertain both in terms of its effectiveness and his ability to tolerate it. Given his psychiatric history he may become acutely psychotic again and withdraw his treatment permission, raising questions about his capacity to consent. Clearly, there are no easy answers here but the commitment of Ahmed's 'team' (enabled by Gary's efforts) promises future shared labours over Ahmed's care.

PALLIATIVE CARE

Sepulveda et al. (2002) noted the global disparity in the provision of effective palliative care and argues that palliation should be considered as soon as it is known that a person is likely to die from their disease. Murray et al. (2005) have described three typical illness trajectories towards death and suggest that cancer typically gives rise to a reasonably predictable decline, thus presenting a context in which quality of life and a 'good death' can be enhanced. Of course, not all cancer deaths are typical and the demarcation between curative treatment efforts and palliation can be uncertain in many cases. However, assuming that a phase of palliative care is explicitly identified, we can consider the role of the mental health practitioner. Effective teamwork with other services remains critical and it is important not to make assumptions based on limited or biased evidence about individual wishes. When asked, most people state a preference to die at home (Munday et al. 2007) but, for example, if your social world is very limited after a lifetime of many acute episodes of psychosis, you might prefer to die in a familiar, institutional place. Advocacy is a key principle and non-person-centred organisational strictures may need to be fought against. Why, for example, should a person not be allowed to die on an acute psychiatric ward if this is where they feel best socially integrated and supported?

In the UK the Gold Standards Framework Centre (GSFC) is leading a national programme to improve palliative care for all (GSFC 2010). Their vision is to enable people to live well until they die. Their aims include organisational systems change and facilitating improved care by all health care practitioners. Such policy initiatives can be used as advocacy resources by mental health practitioners. While some practitioners may not feel entirely comfortable discussing dying with their clients, they will have many interactional skills to draw on and can seek support from palliative care specialists if required.

CONCLUSION

It has been argued that the role of the mental health practitioner is to support and facilitate the care of their client across the cancer trajectory. This does not require sophisticated expertise in the complex and evolving field of oncology but a grasp of some fundamental knowledge about cancer and, most importantly, a willingness to find out more when necessary (see below). The use of case studies has attempted to draw out some key ideas about good practice and to illustrate that these rest on a careful analysis of the impact of the person's mental ill-health on their needs around cancer and vice versa. In short, the mental health practitioner should, first, make it their business to understand what is happening to their patient and to share that understanding with them and their kin within a therapeutic partnership, secondly, to collaborate with different health care colleagues in the client's best interests, and finally to put in place robust support and communication strategies that can usefully adapt to the evolving circumstances.

USEFUL RESOURCES

Information and support materials provided for people with cancer, their loved ones and lay people generally are arguably some of the best health information resources available. They are largely provided by charitable organisations. Some focus on cancer overall, others on specific types of cancer. Access to the internet is hugely advantageous in accessing these resources but many are available in paper form too. Specialist cancer treatment centres often include information facilities. Of course not everybody is computer literate or able to read and write, and this will be a consideration for person-centred care.

At the time of writing in the UK we recommend:

Macmillan Cancer Support – www.macmillan.org.uk
Cancer Research – www.cancerresearchuk.org
National Cancer Institute (USA) – www.cancer.gov
Cancer Buddies Network – www.cancerbuddiesnetwork.org
National Gold Standards (UK) – www.goldstandardsframework.org.uk
This is not intended to be an exhaustive list. Type 'cancer information' into a search engine and you can investigate what you think will be helpful.

7

THE PHYSICAL EFFECTS OF COMMONLY MISUSED SUBSTANCES ON PEOPLE WITH MENTAL HEALTH PROBLEMS

PHIL COOPER AND JANE NEVE

Learning outcomes

By the end of this chapter you should be able to:

- Discuss the most commonly misused substances and their physical impact, including their interactions with prescribed drugs and intoxication effects
- Examine how these issues impact on the physical health of individuals with mental health problems
- Outline the principles of physical health assessment for people with mental health problems and substance misuse
- Consider appropriate treatment interventions aimed at optimising the physical wellbeing of individuals with mental health problems and substance misuse

INTRODUCTION

There has been an increase in the range and availability of licit and illicit substances used in society and in people with mental health problems (European Monitoring Centre for Drugs and Drug Addiction 2010). The relationships between mental health, physical health and substance misuse are complex (Ashcroft 2011). The experience of physical health is inextricably linked to our mental health and vice versa: what is good for you physically is likely to be good for you mentally too and poor physical health negatively affects our mental wellbeing (Department of Health 2011a). People who use illicit substances are more prone to experience mental health problems and people with mental health problems use illicit substances far more than the general population.

The coexistence of a mental health problem together with drug and/or alcohol misuse has been defined as 'dual diagnosis' (Department of Health 2006c). This diagnosis can be applied to individuals whose mental illness and drug or alcohol dependency vary in terms of severity. Figure 7.1 provides a pictorial representation of this.

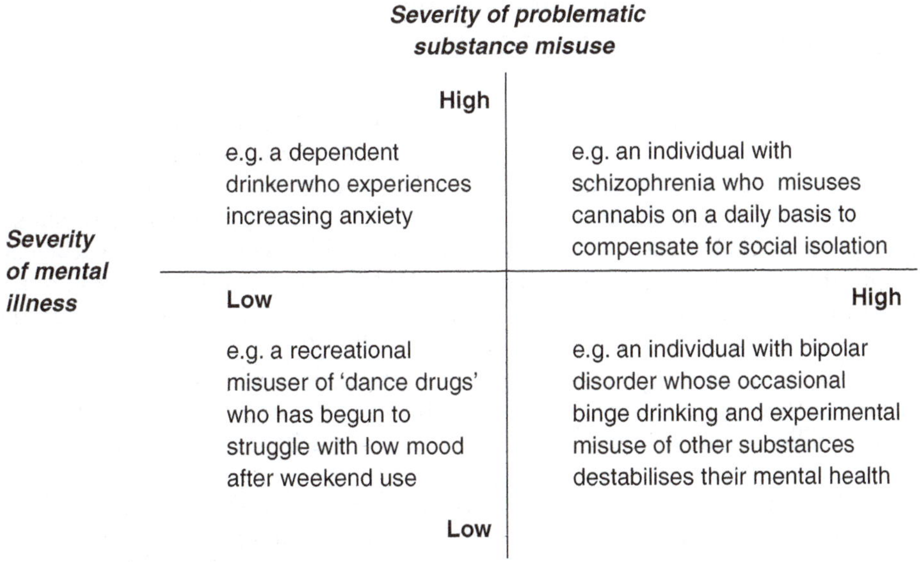

Severity of problematic substance misuse

	High	
Severity of mental illness	e.g. a dependent drinkerwho experiences increasing anxiety	e.g. an individual with schizophrenia who misuses cannabis on a daily basis to compensate for social isolation
	Low	**High**
	e.g. a recreational misuser of 'dance drugs' who has begun to struggle with low mood after weekend use	e.g. an individual with bipolar disorder whose occasional binge drinking and experimental misuse of other substances destabilises their mental health
	Low	

Figure 7.1 The scope of coexistent psychiatric and substance misuse disorders (Department of Health 2002)

In the USA, Drake and Wallach (2000) noted that the concept of dual diagnosis or co-occurring disorders began to emerge during the 1980s and 1990s. Since the early 1990s, the UK government's policy direction has concentrated separately on substance misuse or mental health (Department of Health 2006c). The focus of mental health policy for dual diagnosis was to meet the needs of people with dual diagnosis within mental health services. The separate evolution of mental health from drug and alcohol services meant that mental health workers did not have the skills to assess and treat substance misuse and substance misuse workers did not possess the skills to assess mental health problems. Consequently, service users with a dual diagnosis were passed back and forth between services or tended to fall between service provisions.

The past 20 years have therefore seen clinical and research activity increase in this area, with research focusing on the prevalence of substance misuse among people with a severe mental illness (SMI) and the social and clinical outcomes and interventions that might be effective (National Institute for Health and Clinical Excellence 2010c). The physical health consequences of substance misuse for the individual with a dual diagnosis have received much less attention. This chapter aims to address this gap by shining some further light on the issue.

SUBSTANCE MISUSE AMONG INDIVIDUALS WITH MENTAL HEALTH PROBLEMS

In practically all studies of SMI and substance misuse ('dual diagnosis'), a history of alcohol misuse is most common, followed by either cannabis or cocaine/amphetamine (stimulants) misuse. A very high proportion of service users with psychiatric disorders smoke tobacco (Mueser et al. 2003). Alcohol, cannabis, stimulants and benzodiazepines have been identified by mental health workers as the most common substances used in in-patient mental health settings (Cooper and Evans 2007). Alcohol is the most widely used psychoactive substance in the UK (National Institute for Health and Clinical Excellence 2010b). Alcohol consumption and problems related to alcohol vary widely around the world, but the burden of disease and death remains significant in most countries. The harmful use of alcohol results in approximately 2.5 million deaths each year (World Health Organization 2011).

People with mental health problems are more likely than the general population to use substances (Regier et al. 1990) and dual diagnosis has become far more common in all mental health services, including community, hospital and prison settings (Department of Health 2006c, 2009b).

Dual diagnosis is arguably 'one of the most significant problems facing health services' (McKeown 2010: 3). A significant percentage of general hospital patients are in hospital due to complications relating to alcohol consumption and many people using alcohol or drugs are thought to have mental health problems. Service users with dual diagnosis place considerable demands on health and social care services and are associated with significantly poorer outcomes (see Box 7.1).

> ## Box 7.1 Severity of Problematic Substance Misuse: Outcomes for People with Dual-diagnosis (Department of Health 2002)
>
> Substance misuse among individuals with mental health problems has been associated with significantly poorer outcomes, including:
>
> - Worsening mental health symptoms
> - Increased use of institutional services (community and hospital services)
> - Poor medication adherence
> - Homelessness
> - Increased risk of HIV infection
> - Poor social outcomes, including impact on carers and family
> - Contact with the criminal justice system.

THE PHYSICAL IMPACT OF SUBSTANCE MISUSE

Those with dual diagnosis are at risk of developing physical health problems associated with specific substance administration methods. Just as different drugs have different risks associated with using them, different routes of administration have different risks too. Table 7.1 outlines some of the common ways of taking drugs and some of the associated risks.

Table 7.1 Routes of administration and associated risks

Route of administration	Impact on physical health	Signs and symptoms
Intravenous injection	**Infections** Risk of infection from non-sterile equipment. Cross-infection of blood-borne viruses such as HIV and hepatitis B and C if needles are shared. **Damage to cardiovascular system** Impurities in the solute can lead to blockages in the vessels and even the loss of limbs, deep vein thrombosis and venous irritation. Repeated injections also lead to scarring of the veins and venous collapse.	Signs of localised infection and vascular damage would include: red inflamed skin around injection sites, tracking, cold cyanosed peripheries and painful limbs.

(Continued)

Table 7.1   (Continued)

Route of administration	Impact on physical health	Signs and symptoms
Snorting	Damage to mucus membranes. Necrosis of the septum. Cross-infection from sharing equipment.	Excess mucus is produced causing a runny nose and frequent sniffing. Nose bleeds.
Inhalation	There are more or less dangerous ways of *inhaling* solvents such as glues, gases and aerosols. Squirting solvents into a large plastic bag and then placing the bag over the head has led to death by suffocation. Squirting aerosols or butane straight down the throat has led to deaths through freezing of the airways. Squirting on to a rag or small bag and then inhaling is not as dangerous. The solvent solution also causes irritation to the skin which can lead to infections.	Spots and rash skin around the nose and mouth.
Smoking	The heat, nicotine, tar and impurities in inhaled substances can result in respiratory diseases such as pneumonia, chest infections and lung, mouth and throat cancer.	Frequent coughs, difficulty breathing and/or blood in sputum.
Swallowing	This is a relatively safe method of administration although it can cause tooth decay and irritation of the lining of the digestive system. Synthetic drugs produced for other purposes, such as solvent-based chemicals and poppers, are very dangerous when swallowed, even in small quantities, and may be fatal.	
Suppositories	Very alkaline or acidic substances can lead to burning and damage to the mucus membrane, while the process of inserting suppositories can cause a perforation of the colon.	Rectal bleeding and pain.

In addition, long-term substance misuse can have a devastating and potentially life-threatening effect on bodily systems. To illustrate this, consideration will be afforded to the five most widely used substances among people with mental health problems.

ALCOHOL

Long-term alcohol use can lead to mouth cancer, throat cancer, oesophageal cancer and varices, liver damage, hepatitis, duodenal ulcer, premature ageing, high blood pressure, rapid pulse, anaemia, heart failure, cardiomyopathy, inflammation of the stomach, inflammation of the pancreas, impaired kidney function and reduced fertility (Alcohol Concern 2010).

CANNABIS

Cannabis alters blood flow in the body resulting in dilatation of some blood vessels (which can be seen as redness of the eye) and constriction of others. This can cause higher blood pressure and a strain on the cardiovascular system. Cannabis also increases the heart rate and people with heart problems should avoid its use (Hughes 2010). Risks of use include accidents as a result of lack of concentration and poor reaction times, mental health symptoms triggered or exacerbated, cardiovascular problems, cancer of the mouth, throat and lungs, and lung disease (possibly due to use of tobacco). Cannabis can also make asthma worse, and causes wheezing in non-asthma sufferers (Hussein-Rassool 2010).

Frequent use of cannabis can cut a man's sperm count, reduce sperm motility and can suppress ovulation in women, and so may affect fertility. If pregnant, smoking cannabis frequently may have some association with the risk of the baby being born smaller than expected (Wills 2005).

BENZODIAZEPINES

Benzodiazepines are highly addictive. Tranquillisers are a central nervous system depressant and if taken with other central nervous system depressant drugs, such as alcohol or opiates, can lead to an accidental overdose (Bazire 2007). Some tranquillisers have been shown to cause short-term memory loss. Injecting crushed tablets is extremely dangerous and sometimes fatal. The chalk in tablets is a major cause of collapsed veins which can lead to infection and abscess. Withdrawal can cause unpleasant symptoms, such as a pounding headache, nausea, anxiety and confusion. Some people report withdrawal symptoms after only four weeks' use and withdrawal symptoms can be dangerous and require medical help. Sudden withdrawal after big doses or from some specific drugs can cause panic attacks and fits (Wills 2005).

AMPHETAMINE

Amphetamine puts a strain on the heart and is not advisable for people with hypertension or a heart condition. The combination of amphetamine with antidepressants or alcohol has been known to be fatal. Taking a lot of amphetamine can damage the immune system, resulting in more colds, flu and sore throats. Prepared-for-injection amphetamine may cause vein damage, ulcers and gangrene, especially with dirty needles. Shared needles and injecting equipment can help the spread of viral hepatitis and HIV infections. Injecting amphetamine may be particularly dangerous because it is impure. It is also easier to overdose when injecting (Hussein-Rassool 2010).

COCAINE

Crack and cocaine powder users have died from overdoses. High doses can raise the body's temperature, cause convulsions and respiratory or heart failure. The risk of overdosing increases if crack is mixed with heroin, barbiturates or alcohol. Cocaine is highly risky for anybody with high blood pressure or a heart condition. Perfectly healthy, young people can have a fit or heart attack after taking too much cocaine and the user may not know if they have a pre-existing heart condition. Large or frequent use of cocaine can adversely affect sexual desire, whereas using smaller amounts of cocaine has been associated with increased sexual desire. The same risks of injecting apply to cocaine as well as amphetamine. There is a greater risk of overdose when injecting cocaine. Cocaine is a local anaesthetic and it deadens pain at the injection site, which makes it harder for users to notice the damage they may be doing. Taking cocaine when pregnant can damage the baby. It may cause miscarriage, premature labour and low birth weight. Babies born to mothers who keep using cocaine throughout their pregnancy may experience a withdrawal syndrome after delivery. Regularly smoking crack can cause breathing problems and pains in the chest. Smoking anything damages the lungs (Wills 2005).

Alcohol and cocaine together can be particularly dangerous as the substances interact in the body to produce a toxic chemical (cocaethylene). This interaction produces increased heart rate and blood pressure, increasing the risk of cardiovascular toxicity and liver problems. The risks further increase if other drugs are taken as well. Injecting a mixture of cocaine and heroin, known as 'speedballing', is a dangerous cocktail, with potentially fatal results (Wills 2005).

INTERACTIONS BETWEEN PRESCRIBED MEDICATION AND SUBSTANCES

A further layer of complexity to be considered is the interactions between prescribed psychotropic medication and substances. Bazire (2007) outlines some of these in Table 7.2.

Table 7.2   Interactions between prescribed psychotropic medication and substances (Adapted from Bazire 2007)

Substance	Interactions
Alcohol	Mixing alcohol with prescribed medication can lead to impaired concentration, judgement, coordination, increased drowsiness and lethargy. There is also evidence of enhanced central nervous system depression when combining alcohol and anti-psychotic medication. Low blood pressure and respiratory depression are common interactions and excessive use of alcohol alongside asthma and chest infections could prove fatal. People using alcohol who are prescribed benzodiazepines can experience a more sedative effect of up to 20%–30%.

Substance	Interactions
Cannabis	Increased clearance of Chlorpromazine when a person is smoking cannabis and stopping smoking cannabis can lead to intoxication with Clozapine (if tobacco is used when smoking cannabis). Anti-depressants used with cannabis have been linked to increased heart rate and drowsiness (benzodiazepines). Delirium and mania have been reported with combined Fluoxetine and cannabis use. There is one case of raised lithium levels into the toxic range when using cannabis.
Cocaine	Clozapine can increase cocaine levels, but can reduce the cocaine high and there have been reports of cardiac problems when using cocaine alongside anti-psychotics. Haloperidol may also reduce the stimulant effects of cocaine.

Mental health practitioners need to be aware that service users with an SMI will face a number of physical health dangers (including death) from mixing substances and medication. The evidence relating to interactions with medication of substance misuse can be used as a means to open conversations about substance misuse and potential physical health consequences. Providing objective information that can be challenged by the service user can lead to further discussion that can trigger changes in substance misuse behaviour and improve a service user's mental and physical health. Take a couple of minutes to consider Action Learning Point 7.1.

Action Learning Point 7.1

Taking into account all that you have read so far, identify a client with dual diagnosis and consider the particular risks to their physical health.

THE ROLE OF THE MENTAL HEALTH PRACTITIONER

The role of mental health practitioners is to ensure that the physical health of service users with a dual diagnosis is a priority. Some mental health professionals may perceive their role as only taking care of the dual diagnosis aspects of service users' needs and this may lead to neglect of any related physical health needs (Mears et al. 2001). This perception may be compounded by a feeling that practitioners lack expertise in physical health issues. Choosing to focus narrowly on mental health and substance misuse may particularly be the case in those with a non-nursing background. Friedli and Dardis (2002) have noted that service users attach considerable importance to their physical health but believe that health professionals are predominantly concerned with their mental health problems which they prioritise over their physical health needs. It is the role of the mental health professional to ensure that the physical health needs of service users with a dual diagnosis are seen as a priority, given the overwhelming evidence regarding the negative consequences of failing to address physical health issues (Goldman 1999; Mueser et al. 2003).

Observations by clinicians and service user self-reports have indicated that people with a severe mental health problem typically recover from substance use disorders in a sequence where they become engaged in some type of treatment relationship (Department of Health 2002). People with a dual diagnosis develop motivation to moderate or stop their use of a substance and then adopt active change strategies to attain controlled substance use or, more typically, abstinence. People with a dual diagnosis then endeavour to maintain specific changes and build support networks to prevent relapses. Osher and Kofoed (1989) put forward a four-stage model of the recovery process for consideration. The stages are:

- Engagement
- Persuasion/motivation for change
- Active treatment
- Relapse prevention

While each stage is presented here as a distinct phase, in reality success is dependent upon the interrelationship between each stage. For example, relapse prevention, engagement and assessment of motivation need to be ongoing throughout the whole of the process.

ENGAGEMENT

Mental health professionals can do nothing to enhance the physical, mental or social wellbeing of clients with dual diagnosis unless the individuals decide to engage with service providers. Therefore, the first step towards recovery is to encourage engagement. One approach that can be used to engage service users into treatment can be harm or risk reduction. Harm reduction interventions work to reduce health, social and economic harm to service users (National Treatment Agency 2008). When engaging service users with a dual diagnosis offering clean needles or help with accessing housing support may be more important than medication options and can be used as a starting point for engagement.

Mental health practitioners should subsequently ensure that they place physical health and health promotion at the core of their interventions with service users. They should ensure that service users are included in primary care interventions and are invited for physical health screening. In the UK, for example, primary care services are expected to keep registers of their patients with SMI and proactively screen their health, and mental health practitioners have a big role in facilitating this. Not only should they be proactive in finding out when the screening is due to take place, but they are also in an ideal situation to ascertain if the service user needs support to access the appointment. The service user will need to understand the context of, and the purpose of, the screening and they may have specific concerns about attending, for instance feeling fearful of attending for blood tests if they believe they have put themselves at risk in terms of contracting a blood-borne virus. The practitioner can explore the issues of concern and support the service user using methods such as motivational interviewing. Motivational interviewing is an evidence-based approach to overcoming ambivalence that keeps people from making desired changes (Miller and Rollnick 2002). Mental health teams are additionally encouraged to develop effective relationships with primary care colleagues with the aim of facilitating physical health assessment and treatment to engage service users.

For some service users, screening may have highlighted a plethora of issues that can appear overwhelming and result in reluctance to address problems. Mental health practitioners can guide the service user through this so that agreed priorities can be incorporated into care planning in manageable steps that are appropriate and meaningful. The mental health practitioner is uniquely placed to support the service user to address physical health issues as they may know when motivation to change has shifted. Mental health practitioners maintain an interpersonal process when seeing a service user (the therapeutic relationship). Now review your own practice by completing Action Learning Point 7.2.

Action Learning Point 7.2

- Explore the availability of physical health screening in your local area.
- Consider how you could facilitate your clients to engage with relevant services.

PERSUASION/MOTIVATION TO CHANGE

Motivation is a product of the interaction between the people involved. Motivation for change can be influenced by the interpersonal process and change is facilitated by communicating in a way that can elicit the service user's own understanding of the advantages of change for them (Miller and Rollnick 2002). An example from practice could be where a service user states clearly that they do not want to change their cannabis smoking. The mental health practitioner can provide objective information about the potential effects that cannabis can have on physical and mental health and ask for comments on the information. The mental health practitioner can then ask the service user to write down or state their views of the advantages and disadvantages for change. Using persuasion (a motivational approach) the mental health practitioner 'is a significant determinant of treatment dropout, retention, adherence and outcome' (Miller and Rollnick 2002: 9) and the practitioner can use the working relationship to help view substance use as problematic.

Where service users will not access physical health screening in primary care, this should be documented at review and within care plans. Ongoing attempts should be made to address this with sensitivity and in light of the practitioner's concern for the person's health. The National Institute for Health and Clinical Excellence (2002) recommends that in these circumstances screenings should be undertaken in secondary mental health care.

ACTIVE TREATMENT

Active treatment refers to the situations where a person with a dual diagnosis is motivated to work on issues relating to substance misuse. The goal of the mental health practitioner is to aid a service user to reduce or stop using a substance (Mueser et al. 2003). It may be appropriate and opportune to use an in-patient admission to ensure that a comprehensive examination and screening is conducted. The results of this should be incorporated into care planning and be communicated to primary care.

The Royal College of Psychiatry (2009) stressed the importance of physical examination, health promotion advice (exercise, diet and smoking cessation) and assessment on admission to inpatient services. A comprehensive physical examination can be considered the start of the treatment stage as it is where the service user will be prompted to consider their health behaviours. Where a service user is an in-patient, the assessment should be conducted within 24 hours of admission and this should include a full health review incorporating all current medications, past and present illnesses and current symptoms, health promotion history and details of health screening. When conducting physical health assessment with this group it is useful to specifically consider the physical consequences of the substances they are using and the route of administration. Table 7.3 offers guidelines to structure the assessment process.

Table 7.3   A proposed structure for a physical health assessment

1	To start a dialogue around physical health.
2	To establish current conditions and treatments and family history.
3	Identify risks such as safeguarding children and adults, blood-borne viruses and infections, tissue viability issues, sexual health risks, pregnancy.
4	Assessment of general health.
5	Reassess readiness for change and identify opportunities to intervene.
6	Identification of priorities from the service user's perspective.
7	Positive reinforcement for changes made.
8	Care planning.

When establishing the services user's current conditions and treatments it is also important to gain a detailed history regarding the patterns of substance use. Atakan (2008) suggests that this should include: age at first use, duration of use, amount, type and strength of substance used over a set period of time, preferred method of use and the effect on the individual's physical, mental and social wellbeing. In addition, the individual's subjective experiences of their substance use, what they perceive to be the gains and losses of this use and how this may have changed over time should be explored.

Using physical health screening may be a means to monitor and subsequently build on successes, enabling the service user to further reduce or even abstain from substances. An example may be using changes in liver function blood test results as a means of gauging the amount of damage alcohol is doing to the liver with positive changes being offered as encouragement and reinforcement.

RELAPSE PREVENTION

People with a dual diagnosis may become free of substances and the challenge for the mental health practitioner is then to attempt to prevent relapse back into using substances. A major goal at this stage is encouraging recognition of high-risk situations for using substances again, for example, certain places (bars for alcohol) or certain people (those who use substances). Alongside high-risk situations there are also feelings that are associated with using substances, for example, feeling excited, anxious and guilty and aiming to increase recognition of these can help to prevent the service user from using substances again. Physical health changes or previous problems related to substance misuse can be used to aid a person to recognise the importance of abstinence, thus acting to reinforce this behaviour. Consider Action Learning Point 7.3 and then take a look at the case study of May, which outlines a best practice approach to the physical health needs of a service user with dual diagnosis.

Action Learning Point 7.3

- Consider how you might use your knowledge of the physical impact of substance misuse to aid relapse prevention.
- Identify appropriate health promotion materials to use in relapse prevention and consider devising a resource bank to draw on.

May

May is 34 years old and has a diagnosis of schizophrenia. She has a history of smoking cannabis on a daily basis and of using alcohol (usually strong lager, 5% alcohol by volume (ABV)) to manage persecutory delusional beliefs, auditory hallucinations and severe anxiety symptoms. She rarely leaves the house she shares with her mother except to attend the Clozapine clinic. She has been taking

(Continued)

CASE STUDY

(Continued)

Clozapine for one year and is currently prescribed 450 mgs daily. Her psychotic symptoms have significantly improved and she acknowledges the improvement but is unconvinced of the link between the improvement and the medication. She has abstained from using cannabis almost totally for six months. She currently uses alcohol, approximately three times a week when she drinks approximately five cans of strong lager (5% ABV). May's care team are concerned about her physical health and take the following actions:

- They introduce physical health needs as part of the engagement process and ensure that May is listed on her family doctor's SMI register. They find that an appointment has not yet been made for May to attend for screening.
- They take the opportunity to educate May regarding the physical health impact of her alcohol use, ensuring she understands the implications of continued use.
- They use a motivational approach to discuss any concerns May has about attending physical health screening and, with her permission, arrange for her to attend her family doctor's surgery for a full physical health screen, including a blood test for liver damage (and others).
- They explore the potential interactions between Clozapine and alcohol, again ensuring that May is aware of these and knows how to monitor them.
- They ascertain May's readiness to change her alcohol use and consider what would be the high-risk situations for a relapse should May stop using alcohol.
- They ask how May managed to stop using cannabis (if she has) and consider whether similar strategies might be used in relation to her alcohol use.
- As May rarely leaves her home, they consider how she accesses substances and whether this has any implications in terms of educating her mother.

CONCLUSION

The care of individuals with dual diagnoses is already a complex area of practice in which mental health professionals have to consider their clients' mental health needs alongside their substance misuse. Addressing the physical health needs is yet another complication, but it is a necessary one if we are going to improve the life chances of people with a dual diagnosis.

Achieving this is undoubtedly a challenge, but Osher and Kofoed's (1989) model provides a basis from which we can develop. A starting point is to broaden our engagement with people with dual diagnosis to include physical health screening. Actively motivating them to consider their physical wellbeing is also imperative and should be a consideration throughout. Treatment should start with a holistic assessment which includes the client's physical health (Department of Health 2006c) and the impact on this of repeated substance misuse should be incorporated into relapse prevention strategies. An approach that fails to consider such a model runs the risk of providing ineffective treatment and not only will this fail the service user but it will also fail the mental health practitioner employing it.

USEFUL RESOURCES

At the time of writing in the UK we recommend the following resources:

NICE guidance – www.nice.org.uk
Alcohol Learning Centre – www.alcohollearningcentre.org.uk
National Treatment Agency – www.nta.nhs.uk
Talk to Frank – www.talktofrank.com
Progress National Consortium of Nurse Consultants in Dual Diagnosis – www.dualdiagnosis.co.uk

8

SEXUAL HEALTH IN MENTAL HEALTH PRACTICE

JO BATES

Learning outcomes

By the end of this chapter you should be able to:

- Consider the concept of sexual health
- Identify some of the most prevalent sexually transmitted infections (STIs), including signs and symptoms, treatment and prevention
- Discuss contraceptive methods, including their advantages and disadvantages
- Explore the role of the mental health practitioner in facilitating good sexual health

INTRODUCTION

This chapter will introduce the concept of sexual health and relate this specifically to the needs of clients with mental health problems. Sexual health is a broad, diverse, multifaceted and challenging area of health care and the term 'sexual health' often means different things to different people. Some may immediately think of illness and infections such as sexually transmitted infections (STIs) and human immunodeficiency virus (HIV), whereas others may think of contraception or women's health, including cervical smears and breast screening. Indeed, sexual health does include these topics, but it also includes much more than that.

Sexual health is holistic, involving the whole person in both body and mind and affecting each and every one of us throughout our lifespan, whether we are ill or not.

Good sexual health is essential to good general health and to our sense of wellbeing and quality of life, whether we choose to be sexually active or not. There are many definitions of sexual health and the one below is offered by the Department of Health (DH) (2001: 7):

> Sexual health is an important part of physical and mental health. It is a key part of our identity as human beings together with the fundamental human rights to privacy, a family life and living free from discrimination. Essential elements of good sexual health are equitable relationships and sexual fulfilment with access to information and services to avoid the risk of unintended pregnancy, illness or disease.

While this definition shows the importance of sexual health to our identity, it is focused largely on the prevention of illness, infections and unintended pregnancy. A further definition from the World Health Organization (WHO) (2012) takes a more holistic view in that it sees sexual health as:

> a state of physical, mental and social well-being in relation to sexuality. It requires a positive and respectful approach to sexuality and sexual relationships, as well as the possibility of having pleasurable and safe sexual experiences, free of coercion, discrimination and violence.

Essentially, as stated by Quinn and Browne (2009), sexuality and sexual health are vital components of our life, playing a key role in the overall quality of life and in our general wellbeing. World Association for Sexual Health (1999) go on to advocate that sexual health involves sexual rights that are a basic human given and these are as follows:

- The right to sexual freedom
- The right to sexual autonomy, sexual integrity and safety of the sexual body
- The right to sexual privacy
- The right to sexual equality
- The right to sexual pleasure
- The right to emotional sexual expression
- The right to sexually associate freely
- The right to make free and responsible reproductive choices
- The right to sexual information based on scientific inquiry
- The right to comprehensive sexuality education
- The right to sexual health care

While sexual health is an important aspect of life, it is an issue that is often overlooked in health care practice. Several studies have shown that nurses do not discuss sexual matters with their clients for a variety of reasons, most commonly a lack of knowledge, conservative attitudes, fear of offending clients and embarrassment (McCann 2003; Brown et al. 2008; Matevosyan 2009; Quinn and Browne 2009). Other factors, such as lack of time, fear of being perceived as encouraging sex and the perceived risk of creating emotional turmoil, have also been found to hinder some nurses discussing sexual matters with their clients (Brown et al. 2008). Johnson et al. (2002) add that wider health professionals are also reluctant to discuss sexual issues, largely due to a belief that such matters are personal, thus reinforcing that sexual health is a neglected area of health care.

To compound this, Wakley et al. (2003) report that clients are also reluctant to discuss sexual matters, stating similar reasons to that of health care professionals, such as being embarrassed and feeling ill at ease. In addition, clients state that they feel humiliated, ashamed, are worried about being judged and of having their partner present, unease about their sexuality and concerns about confidentiality. Furthermore, McCann (2003) and Higgins et al. (2006) found that clients are often unaware that their illness or treatment may have consequences in relation to their sexual health, thus suggesting a lack of knowledge that appears currently to be shared with the health professional.

Given the reluctance of both health professionals and clients to discuss sexual health, it is unsurprising that this is a commonly neglected area of practice, but with potentially long-term consequences to both physical and mental health the situation needs to change. It is imperative, therefore, that all health professionals who work with people with mental health disorders feel confident to at least bring up the topic of sexual health with their clients and that they also have a basic knowledge of this sensitive and important area of health care. Being an expert is not a requirement of addressing this topic; indeed, taking that first step of initiating a discussion could well make all the difference. Before going further, consider the issues raised in Action Learning Point 8.1.

Action Learning Point 8.1

Consider the following;

- Do you talk to clients/patients about sexual health issues?
- If not what stops you?
- What level of knowledge do you have in relation to sexual health?
- Do you need to develop this knowledge further?

SEXUAL HEALTH AND INDIVIDUALS WITH MENTAL HEALTH PROBLEMS

There is evidence to suggest that individuals with mental health problems are at an increased risk of poorer sexual health when compared with the general population. In particular, the risk of contracting STIs and HIV is higher than in the general population, as is the possibility of having an unintended pregnancy (Rosenberg et al. 2001; Brown et al. 2006; Carey et al. 2007; Brown et al. 2008; and Matevosyan 2009).

According to Farr et al. (2010), 20% of women with mental distress do not use contraception, or when they do, they use contraception that is less effective. An unfortunate consequence of unintended pregnancy in a woman with a mental health disorder is a potential worsening of their condition, resulting in adverse outcomes for both mother and baby (Farr et al. 2010). In relation to STIs, research by Matevosyan (2009) showed that 34% of patients with an STI also had a co-morbid mental health disorder. While both of these studies were conducted in the USA, and may not therefore be generalised to other countries or populations, it certainly presents food for thought.

Chronic illnesses, which include many of the mental health disorders, can also have a significant impact on an individual's (and consequently their partner's) sexual health as these affect libido, self-image and general physical and psychological wellbeing. This in turn can influence decision-making and choice (Warner et al. 1999). An example is the documented assertion that people with a mental health disorder are more likely to engage in risk-taking behaviour such as having sex at a young age, having unprotected sex, engaging multiple partners who may themselves be in a high-risk group, injecting drug use and sex trading (Rosenberg et al. 2001; Brown et al. 2008; Quinn and Brown 2009).

There are also further considerations in relation to the vulnerability of individuals with a mental health problem, starting with the proposal that they are at increased risk of experiencing periods of homelessness, social disadvantage and poverty, all lifestyle issues that can add to their potential for vulnerability to sexual health problems (Drake et al. 1991; Berkman and Kawachi 2000; Carey et al. 2007). Treatment for mental health disorders can also cause side-effects linked to sexual dysfunction and, conversely, the condition itself may cause an array of sexual problems, all of which impact on general health and wellbeing, but more specifically on sexual health and wellbeing.

SEXUALLY TRANSMITTED INFECTIONS (STIs)

STIs are infections contracted via sexual contact with another person and are caused by bacteria, viruses or protozoa. The long-term consequences of undiagnosed and untreated STIs are serious and sometimes fatal, and they present a major public health problem in the world today (Adler 2004). STIs have been known about for centuries, with some well-known individuals from history acquiring STIs. Today STIs are still often associated with stigma and shame because of the nature of how they are contracted and this stigma can present a huge barrier to individuals accessing treatment (Bannerman and Proom 2009). Additionally, the risk of contracting an STI or HIV is linked with the type of sexual activity and number of partners, and the risk increases the more sexual partners a person has (Wakley et al. 2003). However, it is important to recognise that an individual may only have sexual contact with one person but if that person has an STI or HIV then there is the potential for cross-infection. Remember that not everyone with an STI has had sexual contact with multiple partners.

The long-term consequences of untreated STIs can be devastating. Chlamydia, for example, may be asymptomatic but can result in symptoms such inter-menstrual bleeding and pelvic inflammatory disease in women, which in turn can cause ectopic pregnancies and infertility. In men, the infection may result in urethral discharge, proctitis, conjunctivitis and reactive arthritis (Richens 2004). The World Health Organization (2000) describe STIs as falling into one of four groups:

- Viral infections (including HIV, acquired immune deficiency syndrome (AIDS), herpes simplex 1 and 2, human papilloma virus (HPV), hepatitis B and others)
- Bacterial infections (including chlamydia, syphilis, gonorrhoea, trichomonas, gardenerella and others)
- Yeast infections (including candidiasis and others)
- Infestations (including pubic crabs, scabies and others).

An understanding of the common STIs, routes of transmission and signs and symptoms is invaluable for health care professionals.
- Chlamydia – The most commonly diagnosed STI in young men (age 20–24) and women (age 16–19) in England, Wales and Northern Ireland. It can be transmitted from one mucous membrane to another, e.g. throat, eyes and anus, by close physical contact. Chlamydia can also be transmitted from mother to baby during labour.

  Signs and symptoms: Asymptomatic in up to 80% of women and 50% of men; women may also experience post-coital bleeding, inter-menstrual bleeding, vaginal discharge, pelvic inflammatory disease; both genders may experience genital inflammation and swelling, sore throat, pain on urination and lower abdominal pain.
  Treatment: Oral antibiotics

- Gonorrhoea – Transmitted by close physical contact from one mucous membrane to another. Easily transmitted via vaginal, oral and anal sex. Can be transmitted from mother to baby.

  Signs and symptoms: Up to 50% of cases in women and 10% in men will be asymptomatic; symptoms include genital discharge, lower abdominal pain and pain on urination.
  Treatment: Oral antibiotics

- Syphilis – The primary route of transmission is via sexual contact but syphilis can also be transmitted from mother to child. If untreated, it leads to a systemic disease with a variety of clinical complications which over time may be fatal.

  Signs and symptoms: Painless ulcer (chancre) at site of exposure (usually genitals, perianal area or mouth), skin rash and systemic illness.
  Treatment: Treated with antibiotics via intramuscular (IM) injection preferably, but can be treated with oral antibiotics.

- HIV – Viral infection transmitted via sexual contact, blood to blood (e.g. needlestick injury or infected blood products being transfused), mother to baby. It can take up to three months for antibodies to appear in the blood following infection with the virus. This is called the 'window period'. Testing for HIV antibodies should therefore take place at time of exposure and then be repeated three months later.

Signs and symptoms: Upon initial infection the following signs and symptoms may occur (although they often go unnoticed or are put down to having a cold or feeling 'off colour' as most people will recover within 2–4 weeks): high temperature, fatigue, skin rash, myalgia, headaches, sore throat, mouth ulcers, swollen lymph glands, nausea, diarrhoea, weight loss, night sweats, oral thrush, cough (not an exhaustive list). If the virus remains undetected (many people will be asymptomatic), it will over a period of time start to damage the immune system of the infected person. They will then become susceptible to infections such as oral thrush, vaginal thrush, gastro-intestinal infections resulting in diarrhoea, pulmonary infections, herpes simplex infections, skin cancer and pneumonia (not an exhaustive list).

Treatment: At this point in time there is no cure for HIV or AIDS, although modern drug treatments have greatly improved both the quality and length of life for those infected with the virus.

- Genital warts – Many types of warts have been detected (over 100) and they are caused by the human papilloma virus (HPV). Certain strains cause genital and perianal warts, and some strains have been associated with cervical cancer.

  Signs and symptoms: Single or multiple fleshy growths which are painless and may or may not be itchy; can cause psychological distress as they may reoccur.
  Treatment: Various treatments available.

- Genital herpes (herpes simplex virus HSV) – HSV 1 usually affects the lips and mouth area. HSV 2 usually affects the ano-genital area. It is, however, possible to transfer both types so that HSV 1 is found in the genital area and HSV 2 is found in the mouth and lips. Transmitted by skin-to-skin contact with a herpes lesion (blister), such as during kissing, oral sex or other sexual contact. Mother to baby transmission can occur.

  Signs and symptoms: For both men and women the infection may cause tingling, burning or itching sensation; small fluid filled blisters appear at the site of infection which are very painful; in the genital region the blister may make passing urine painful, sometimes resulting in urinary retention which requires catheterisation and hospital admission; can cause pyrexia and myalgia and flu-like symptoms.
  Treatment: Various treatments for the symptoms are available and analgesia may also be required during an outbreak.

- Hepatitis B – Can be transmitted by sexual contact, via blood and blood products and from mother to baby.
  Signs and symptoms: May be asymptomatic in the acute phase for some people; can cause flu-like symptoms, lethargy, diarrhoea, fever, loss of appetite and weight loss, nausea and vomiting, jaundice of the skin, itchy skin, upper right-sided abdominal pain.
  Treatment: Referral to a doctor is required for monitoring of the condition. Immunisation against the infection is available.

- Hepatitis C – Transmitted via IV drug use, infected blood and blood products, body piercing and tattoos with unclean needles. Transmission via sexual activity and from mother to baby carries a lower risk.

  Signs and symptoms: Over 80% of people are asymptomatic but the following may occur: tiredness, nausea.

  Treatment: Referral to a doctor is required for monitoring of the condition. No immunisation is currently available (Richens 2004; Peate 2005; Bannerman and Proom 2009).

THE ROLE OF THE MENTAL HEALTH PRACTITIONER

Appropriate awareness and knowledge of sexual health are a prerequisite of quality care for people with mental health problems. Strategies include the incorporation of sexual health within a systematic physical health assessment (discussed further in Chapter 2) and the promotion of effective contraception and safer sex.

SEXUAL HEALTH ASSESSMENT

The most important thing that a mental health professional can do to enhance the sexual wellbeing of their clients is to engage them in a discussion regarding their sexual health. It is imperative not to stereotype people according to race, gender, sexual activity, age or illness, but to assess each person's risk on an individual basis. While mental health practitioners are well versed in communication and engagement strategies, they are unlikely to feel equipped to discuss sexual health issues as few health professionals receive training in this potentially delicate art. The core skills, however, remain unchanged and so mental health professionals should feel confident in employing their existing proficiency in relationship development and complement these with some key prompt questions specifically focused on sexual health.

If the discussion is part of a formal assessment, it may feel more comfortable to tell the client that sexual health is part of the holistic approach and that the questions that are about to be asked are standard for everybody. To break the ice, asking whether the client is in a sexual relationship currently can be a good starting point, followed by enquiring whether they, or their partner, are having any sexual difficulties. If the client appears willing to discuss this, then asking whether they are satisfied with their sex life and whether they have any sexual concerns they would like to discuss are good open questions that can elicit information and encourage discussion. Once the client has started to open up, the aim will be to take a fuller sexual history with a question such as 'Would you mind telling me about your sexual history?' With an added prompt such as 'Perhaps your first sexual experience?' or

'Could you tell me how many partners you've had?' This may identify negative and/ or abusive experiences and, while the mental health practitioner should be aware of and sensitive to this, it does not have to negate continuing with the assessment. Instead, clinical judgement will need to be applied.

When taking a sexual history it is important to consider both past and present circumstances and questions should be aimed at identifying sexual behaviours and orientation, sexual difficulties or concerns, sexually transmitted diseases, contraception methods and alcohol and drug use (prescribed and recreational). Whether safe sex has and is still being practised is a key area for exploration and an excellent lead into the promotion of sex education.

Where the discussion of sexual health falls outside a formal assessment, perhaps in a routine visit or a conversation on a ward, the practitioner may want to think about initiating the conversation by asking clients how they are finding their medication and whether they have experienced any disruption to their sexual functioning as a result. Similarly, where clients are using drugs or alcohol, it may be appropriate to ask if these have had any impact on their experience or behaviour in relation to sex. In both situations the fact that sexual ill-health can be a consequence can provide a rationale to the client for initiating the conversation, which will also help normalise anything the client may wish to raise.

Many STIs have common presenting signs and symptoms which should act as a trigger to indicate that a client should be advised to attend a sexual health screening unit. There is no suggestion that mental health professionals conduct physical examinations; rather, they are encouraged to be attuned to the cues that may indicate a need for referral. These cues could include vaginal discharge and possibly (but not always) vaginal discomfort and irritation, genital ulceration and urethral discharge (Adler 2004). Discharge from the penis in men is abnormal and requires further investigation, whereas in women some vaginal discharge is normal. However, if the vaginal discharge becomes offensive in smell, itchy, more purulent or changes from what is considered normal by the woman, this will require further investigation (Bannerman and Proom 2009). It is helpful to remember that in many cases STIs co-exist together so if a person is infected with one STI, they will need to be fully screened as it may be that they are also infected with another STI as well.

SEXUAL HEALTH PROMOTION AND CONTRACEPTION

Health promotion is an important part of any health professional's role. Indeed, professionals will be familiar with the Ottawa Charter, which states that 'Health promotion is the process of enabling people to increase control over and to improve their health' (World Health Organization 1986: 1).

This is an apt definition when considering the purpose of sexual health promotion. Ultimately, the aim is to equip individuals with knowledge and skills to take control over the sexual health choices they make. This should be delivered in a non-judgemental and supportive way by health professionals who have at least a basic understanding of sexual health matters, have the ability to communicate effectively with others and be self-aware (Ingram-Fogel 1990, cited in Rowe et al. 2009). The latter is particularly important given the wide array of sexual preferences in terms of sexuality and sexual behaviours (promiscuity, fetishes) which you may encounter. In order to enhance your own self-awareness, it is therefore important that you take some time to consider your beliefs and values and Action Learning Point 8.2 will assist with this.

Action Learning Point 8.2

- Do you have any strongly held beliefs and values about sex and sexual behaviour?
- If so, what are these and how did you come to hold these beliefs?
- Do you make assumptions about a person's sexual identity and sexual preference?

Most of us tend to assume that most people are heterosexual or 'straight' when in fact this may not be the case. Burrows (2011) states that in the UK it is estimated that between 0.3% and 10% of the population report as being lesbian, gay or bisexual (LGB). Indeed, people who are LGB suffer health inequalities due to factors such as social exclusion, inappropriately designed services and lack of awareness among health professionals (Burrows 2011). When considering people with mental health problems this is likely to be compounded even more. A small way in which a difference can be made in relation to becoming more inclusive is to consider the language you use. For example, when dealing with a woman do you refer to her husband? If so, unless you know otherwise, this is making assumptions. First, does the woman have a partner or is she single? Second, if she does have a partner is that person male or female? Try to use words such as 'your partner'. If assumptions are made about a person's sexuality and sexual preferences it is very difficult for them to correct that assumption as they may be unsure and even fearful of the reaction and response they may get.

When promoting sexual health with clients it is also extremely important that the mental health practitioner is able to be non-judgemental. To do so you may need to put aside your beliefs and values and focus on maximising the sexual wellbeing of your client. This may not be easy and can cause emotional conflict for some. If this is the case for you, then you should seek help and support yourself in order that you can resolve any personal issues to enable you to work more effectively in your professional role.

Encouraging men and women to use an effective method of contraception, facilitating access to contraception and contraceptive services is an extremely important part of sexual health care. This has the dual aim of protecting against STIs and preventing unplanned pregnancies, thus enabling people to choose when and if to reproduce.

There are many factors to consider when advising about contraception for women with a mental health disorder. For example, St Johns' Wort is a herbal preparation available in many pharmacies, chemists and herbal stores and is used to help alleviate low mood. However, it can interfere with the Combined Oral Contraceptive pill (COC) commonly known as 'the pill' and the Progestogen Only Pill (POP), commonly known as the 'mini pill', potentially affecting their efficacy (Guillebaud and Macgregor 2009; Glasier and Gebbie 2008; Bekaert and White 2006). Break through bleeding (BTB), or spotting bleeding as it is sometimes called, can be a disadvantage of progestogen-only methods of contraception such as the mini pill and Depo Provera, and this may not be well tolerated in some women with a mental health disorder (Matevosyan 2009). When considering contraception it is important to note that only condoms protect against the transmission of STIs and HIV, and only if they are used correctly each time the person has sex. Therefore health professionals should take the opportunity to discuss the use of condoms even if the person is using a hormonal method of contraception such as the COC. The hormonal method will protect against unintended pregnancy and condoms will protect against STIs and HIV.

There are a range of Medical Eligibility Criteria (MEC) developed by the World Health Organization (2012) to assist and guide health professionals when advising and prescribing methods of contraception (2012). Contraceptive methods are categorised according to the presence of specific illnesses or conditions. Contraception is considered in terms of whether the advantages of using the method outweigh the risks of taking it. Those eligible should not have a condition for which there is a restriction for the use of the contraceptive method, or the theoretical or proven risks usually outweigh the advantages of using the method. The contraceptive method should not be used if this represents an unacceptable health risk or where the advantages of using the method generally outweigh the theoretical or proven risks (WHO 2012). In the UK, they have been adopted and adapted by the Faculty of Family Planning and Reproductive Health Care in 2006 and are referred to as the UKMEC (French 2009).

Mental health practitioners cannot be expected to be expert in contraception, but it is helpful to have a basic understanding of the contraceptive methods available and their advantages and disadvantages. It is important that you encourage both men and women to seek expert advice, especially if they are taking any form of medication and/or have any medical conditions. Table 8.1 outlines common contraceptive methods and their advantages and disadvantages. It is also important to reiterate that the majority of contraceptive devices do not protect against STIs and, as such, clients should always be advised to use condoms in addition to their chosen method of contraception.

Table 8.1 Common contraceptive methods

Contraceptive method	Advantages	Disadvantages
Male condom 85–98% effective	Widely and easily available The only contraceptive method that protects against STIs and HIV when used correctly and consistently. Available over the counter or via the internet. Available in various colours, flavours, sizes, etc. There are no medical side effects.	Some people say it interferes with the spontaneity of sex and some men report feelings of reduced sensation. Latex sensitivity can occur – alternative non-latex condoms must be used for people with a latex allergy.
Female condom 79–95% effective	Reduced sensation is less likely for the male. An effective method that is controlled by the woman. Available over the counter or via the internet. Protects against STIs. Made of strong polyurethane so there is reduced risk of splitting when compared with the male condom.	Not suitable for women who dislike touching their genitalia. Unattractive appearance. Can be noisy during sex. Penetration can sometimes occur outside the condom and sometimes the condom may be pushed up into the vagina.
Diaphragm 84–94% effective	Woman controlled. Can be used by women who are breastfeeding. Spermicide use provides additional vaginal lubrication. Gives some protection against pelvic inflammatory disease. Gives protection against pre-malignant disease and carcinoma of the cervix. Reusable. Can be inserted up to several hours before intercourse. No hormonal side-effects.	Latex sensitivity can occur. Risk of toxic shock syndrome if the diaphragm is left *in situ* over a prolonged period. Not suitable for women who dislike touching their genitalia. Needs to be refitted if the woman gains or loses 7lbs of weight and also following childbirth and pelvic surgery. Requires insertion before intercourse. Spermicide can be messy. Initial fitting must be carried out by a trained doctor or nurse. Does not protect against STIs and HIV. May cause some loss of sensation for the woman and also some discomfort. Increased risk of urinary tract infections. Must be motivated to continue using this method.
Combined Oral Contraceptive pill (COC), commonly	Highly effective if taken correctly and consistently. Regulates menstruation so periods can be predicted.	**Not suitable for all women therefore expert advice should be sought** Does not protect against STIs and HIV.

Contraceptive method	Advantages	Disadvantages
known as the pill, 92–99% effective	Reduces PMT symptoms, bleeding and menstrual pain. Provides protection against ovarian, endometrial and bowel cancer. Reduces ovarian cysts. Nearly 100% reversible. Does not interfere with sex.	Side-effects can include: break through bleeding (BTB) or 'spotting' bleeding, nausea, breast tenderness and mood changes, headaches, migraines, weight gain, depression, reduced libido. Efficacy may be affected by some medicines such as St John's Wort, some anticonvulsants, some antibiotics and some antiretrovirals. There may be a slight increase in risk of breast cancer, although this is uncertain. There may be an increased risk of thrombosis and stroke for some women – this risk increases if the woman smokes and is over 35 years old. Long-term use of the COC (over 8 years) may slightly increase the risk of cervical cancer.
Progestogen Only Pill (POP) commonly known as 'the mini pill' 96–99% efficacy with consistent use	Does not contain oestrogen and may therefore be suitable for women who are unable to take the COC. Effective method of contraception if taken correctly and consistently. Can be used by women who are breastfeeding. Does not interfere with sex.	**Although the POP is very safe, there are a few women for whom the POP is not suitable, therefore expert advice should be sought** Must be taken within a 3-hour margin every 24 hours (Cerazette 12-hour margin). Ovarian cysts and risk of ectopic pregnancy in conception does occur. Some women report weight gain, acne, breast tenderness, spotting, bleeding and erratic bleeding patterns. Does not protect against STIs and HIV.
Progestogen only injection (Long-Acting Reversible Contraception [LARC]) 99–100% efficacy	Highly effective method of contraception. Does not contain oestrogen and may therefore be suitable for women who are unable to take the COC. Does not interfere with sex. Need to have a repeat injection every 12 weeks so do not have to remember to take a pill daily Protects against pelvic infection and cancer of the uterus. Not affected by other medicines.	**Not suitable for all women therefore expert advice should be sought** Have to wait at least 12 weeks for the effects of the injection to subside. Need to return to health provider for repeat injection every 12 weeks. Reported side-effects include weight gain, spotting, irregular bleeding, mood changes, breast tenderness and loss of libido. Delay in return of fertility from a few months up to 18 months on stopping the injection.

(Continued)

Table 8.1   (Continued)

Contraceptive method	Advantages	Disadvantages
	Can be used by women who are breastfeeding. Some women will have no bleeding which can be seen as an advantage.	Does not protect against STIs and HIV. There is a possible link between the progestogen injection and an increased risk of osteoporosis.
Intra-Uterine System (IUS) known as the Mirena Coil and **Intra-Uterine Device (IUD)** commonly known as 'the coil') Both methods are LARCs 97–99% efficacy	Both devices are highly effective methods of contraception. Long-lasting between three and five years depending on device used. Does not interfere with sex. Can be used by women who are breastfeeding. Does not contain oestrogen and therefore may be suitable for women who are unable to take the COC. Fully reversible on removal. Mirena coil can be used to treat heavy and painful periods.	Needs insertion by a qualified doctor or nurse. Insertion may be uncomfortable for some women. Small risk of uterine perforation. The IUD may increase menstrual blood loss. There may be some progestogen side-effects with the Mirena coil, such as spotting bleeding. Does not protect against STIs and HIV.
Progestogen implant known as Implanon and Nexplanon Efficacy >99% It is a LARC method	Highly effective method of contraception. Long-acting (three years). Fully reversible on removal Does not contain oestrogen and may therefore be suitable for women who are unable to take the COC. Does not interfere with sex. Can be used by women who are breastfeeding after six weeks following the birth. No evidence that it affects bone mineral density.	Needs insertion and removal by a qualified doctor or nurse. Small risk of complications following insertion, such as infection, bruising, bleeding and scarring. Sometimes may be difficult to remove. Possible side-effects, including weight gain, headaches, breast tenderness, altered bleeding pattern, such as spotting bleeding. Does not protect against STIs and HIV.
Emergency contraception 'the morning after pill' (pill containing progestogen; only known as Levonelle in the UK)	Safe method for when other methods have not been taken correctly or not used.	Can cause nausea and vomiting. Does not protect against STIs and HIV. May alter bleeding pattern.

Before moving on to the conclusion, utilise the information from this chapter to consider the following case study.

Clara

Clara is a 34 year-old married lady who works part-time as a clerical worker and has two young children. She was diagnosed with manic depression in her early twenties but despite having had long periods of remission she has also had several short but intense periods of mania, some of which have led to brief hospital admissions. Clara has recently experienced her most severe period of mania yet, and during your visit to her home today she has become very upset. Clara explains that during this period she stayed away from home for five nights with people she had recently met at a party. She is distraught as she recalls that she was highly promiscuous during this time and had sexual encounters with a number of different men. Clara's primary concern is the potential damage this may do to her marriage and she is struggling to decide what to disclose to her husband. She rebuffs your suggestion that she visit her GP or sexual health centre as she feels embarrassed.

- What are the risks to Clara's sexual health?
- Identify the steps you could take to ensure she receives the optimum care at this time?

Answer guide:

1 Clara is at risk of having contracted an STI. The long-term consequences of undiagnosed and untreated STIs are serious and sometimes fatal, so it is vital that any STI is diagnosed and treated as soon as possible. In addition, Clara is of child-bearing age and there is a risk that she may be pregnant.

2 It is vitally important that you, as her mental health practitioner, are open and willing to discuss this sensitive issue with Clara and every attempt should be made to encourage her to attend a sexual health screening clinic. This may be achieved by highlighting the anonymity of the service, educating her about the importance of early diagnosis and the availability of effective treatments for many infectious conditions, facilitating access and possibly even accompanying her on her visit. However, if this is unsuccessful, then you could assess Clara for the presence of common signs and symptoms of an STI, such as inter-menstrual bleeding, vaginal discharge, genital inflammation and swelling, vaginal ulceration or rash, genital itching, pain on urination and lower abdominal pain. In addition, Clara should be encouraged to take a pregnancy test and may benefit from having the details of a pregnancy advisory service. She should also be strongly encouraged to use a barrier method of contraception until an STI has been ruled out so that she does not risk passing an infection on to her husband. Clara should be made aware of the how to access a sexual health screening service in case she changes her mind at a later date. Lastly, it may be possible to liaise with Clara's family GP, with her consent, to consider the possibility of Clara taking a course of broad-spectrum antibiotics.

CONCLUSION

Good sexual health is a basic human given yet so many people fail to experience this. Both body and mind can be affected by sexual ill-health, yet it is an often over-looked aspect of health care practice. While a variety of reasons have been offered for this, reluctance on the part of the health professional is undoubtedly key, with personal discomfort and a lack of knowledge being at the core of the problem. Addressing this reluctance must, however, be a priority for mental health practitioners as the increased risk of sexual ill-health to individuals with mental health problems adds yet another vulnerability to an already disadvantaged group. By promoting sexual wellbeing, mental health practitioners have the opportunity to enhance the overall health of their clients, while being attuned to the signs of sexual ill-health will facilitate access to appropriate sexual health services.

USEFUL RESOURCES

At the time of writing in the UK we recommend the following resources:

World Health Organization – www.who.int/
HIV and Aids information – www.avert.org.uk
Marie Stopes International – www.mariestopes.org.uk
International Planned Parenthood Federation – www.ippf.org/en

WOUND CARE IN MENTAL HEALTH PRACTICE

LOUISE SHORNEY AND RICHARD SHORNEY

Learning outcomes:

By the end of this chapter you should be able to:

- Describe the anatomy and physiology of the skin and the process of wound healing
- Demonstrate knowledge of wound assessment strategies
- Discuss the management of acute and chronic wounds
- Consider the care of individuals with pressure ulcers and those who self-harm

---

INTRODUCTION

Wound care is a central aspect of nursing practice and is an area that is growing in complexity and sophistication. However, the key principles of wound care management remain unchanged and all health care professionals would benefit from a basic understanding of these principles.

Mental health practitioners often encounter service users with a variety of wounds but, as with the other physical health needs identified within this book, the management of these tends to be a low priority (Nash 2005). Indeed, the report from the Royal College of Psychiatrists (RCP) on physical health in mental health states quite clearly that the predominant view of mental health professionals is that 'physical healthcare is in the province of other clinicians' (RCP 2009: 9), thus their call for a change in practice. Theirs is only one of a growing number of voices emphasising the need to ensure that there is an increased level of competence in the prevention, detection and treatment of general health problems in people with mental health disorders (Department of Health 2005b, 2006a, 2006b; RCP 2009) and thus this chapter aims to assist the development of competence in the area of wound care. More specifically, the chapter will focus on two main areas of wound care: acute wounds commonly encountered when service users have engaged in self-cutting (a form of self-harm) and chronic wounds presenting as pressure ulcers, most typically, though not exclusively, seen in the care of older adults. The reasons for this will be explored below.

WOUND CARE IN MENTAL HEALTH PRACTICE

Self-harm is an area that has received a lot of attention over recent years; partly due to its prevalence among the general population and partly due to the sometimes controversial ways in which individuals who self-injure are managed. In relation to the former, it is reported that between 4% and 6% of people in England have at some point engaged in self-harm behaviour and it is also known to be prevalent in other countries around the world (Hawton et al. 2006). Further, there is general agreement that the reported figures are an underestimation as it is recognised that many acts of self-harm never come to the attention of health care services (Meltzer et al. 2002). Of those who present at accident and emergency services (A&E), it is estimated that a fifth are there as a result of self-inflicted cutting (Horrocks et al. 2003).

While self-harm can occur in all sections of the population, there is a strong association with mental health problems. Hawton et al. (2006) found that most of the attendees at A&E who had self-harmed met the criteria for at least one mental health condition, while Meltzer et al. (2002) state that individuals with a mental health problem are 20% more likely to harm themselves than the general population. Those with schizophrenia are at most risk, with an estimated 50% of such individuals having self-harmed at some point during their illness (Meltzer et al. 2002). The chances of mental health practitioners encountering a self-inflicted wound are therefore high. Although an abundance of literature on the management of self-harm has emerged over recent years, in a bid to move away from the controversial methods employed (no analgesia and punitive practice), it has tended to focus on psychological rather than physical interventions. National Institute for Health and Clinical Excellence (NICE) guidelines published in 2004 recommend that the physical consequences of self-harm be addressed and that staff have the necessary skills to care adequately for individuals who self-harm (NICE 2004b). It would therefore stand to reason that mental health practitioners (MHPs), who are well versed in the psychological aspects of self-harm, focus their development on those aspects that are physical.

Pressure ulcers are also a growing concern globally, particularly in the older adult population, which, due to advances in health technology, is the fastest growing section of the total population (Buck et al. 2009). In England alone it has been estimated that one in 23 of the over-65 population will develop this type of chronic wound (Havard and Western 2007). The older adult population make up a significant proportion of mental health service users and, as such, it is highly likely that MHPs will encounter this type of wound. In the UK the treatment of pressure ulcers causes a financial burden for the National Health Service (NHS) with an estimated 4% of the entire budget being spent on this (Bennett et al. 2004). It is recommended, therefore, that the existence of such wounds should be diagnosed and managed quickly (Buck et al. 2009) and this chapter aims to equip the MHP with the knowledge required to assist in this process.

Although pressure ulcers are seen most predominantly in the older adult group, there is also a risk of these wounds with people of all ages who are obese or who suffer diabetes, both of which are identified elsewhere in the book as potential risk factors for individuals with mental health problems. Indeed, the general poor health and lifestyle choices of such individuals increases both the likelihood of a wound being experienced and of that wound not healing well, which, as a consequence, increases the chance of MHPs encountering the same occurrences. There is therefore a need for MHPs to be clinically equipped to manage these when they present. Thus the overall aim of this chapter is to offer the reader an understanding of the key principles of wound care in order that they can apply it to their field of practice.

STRUCTURE AND FUNCTION OF THE SKIN

The skin's main function is protective; this is achieved by preventing the loss of fluids and electrolytes and inhibiting the penetration of harmful substances. The skin also protects us from injury and changes in temperature, as well as the harmful effects of the environment (Bale and Jones 2006). The regulation of body temperature is an additional function of the skin which is achieved by directing blood flow to or away from the surface to manage heat loss. The skin also conveys mood changes through the colour of the cheeks which can act as an indicator of our physical wellbeing (Timmons 2005).

Often referred to as the largest organ in the body, the skin is comprised of two principal layers, the epidermis and dermis (Timmons 2005). Beneath the dermis is a subcutaneous layer, which consists of connective and adipose tissue.

THE EPIDERMIS

The epidermis is the thin outer layer of the skin which is composed of multiple layers of epithelial cells. These divide at the bottom layer, the Stratum Basale, and push already formed cells into higher layers. As the cells move into the higher layers, they flatten and eventually die. The top layer of the epidermis, the Stratum Corneum, is made of dead, flat skin cells that shed about every two weeks (see Table 9.1).

Table 9.1   Layers of the epidermis

Layers of epidermis	Function
Stratum Corneum	Tough, waterproof, uppermost layer of the epidermis consisting of dead fibrous cells which contain keratin. Keratin helps to waterproof, protect the skin and underlying tissues from heat, light, microbes and chemicals.
Stratum Lucidum	A transparent layer which is thought to provide extra protection as it is present on the palms of the hand and soles of the feet, which are prone to wear and tear.
Stratum Granulosum	This is the layer in which the cells lose their moisture and keratin deposits build up, strengthening the cells and adding water resistance.
Stratum Spionosum	This layer contains desmosomes which 'stick' the cells together and assist in maintaining the integrity of the epidermis.
Stratum Basale	The lowest layer of the epidermis, which forms a border between the dermis and epidermis. The basal cells constantly divide, allowing the continuous regeneration of the skin. Melanocytes are present and they make melanin, the substance which determines skin pigmentation.

THE DERMIS

The dermis is the thickest layer of the skin which sits beneath the epidermis and ranges in thickness from 2 mm to 4 mm. The dermis is composed of connective tissue which contains collagen and elastin fibres, making the structure strong and flexible. Collagen is a protein which gives the skin its tensile strength. This ability declines with age which shows in the formation of wrinkles as the skin loses some of its supporting structure (Timmons 2005).

There are several structures within the dermis and these are outlined in Table 9.2.

Table 9.2   Structures within the dermis

Structure	Function
Blood vessels	Supply oxygen and nutrients to sweat glands and the dermis.
Lymphatic vessels	Responsible for transporting particulate matter and lymphatic fluid away from the dermis.
Sensory nerve endings	Responsible for our sense of touch, temperature and pain.
Sweat glands	*Eccrine* sweat glands are distributed throughout the skin but are most concentrated on the palms and soles. *Apocrine* sweat glands are found mainly in the pubic region, axilla and areolae of the breast. They play a role in the regulation of body temperature.

Structure	Function
Hair	Hair follicles are formed in the dermis but grow through the epidermis.
Arrector pilli muscles	This smooth muscle fibre is attached to the hair follicle and contracts under stress to pull the hairs vertically which traps air close to the skin and retains heat.
Sebaceous glands	Secrete an oily substance called sebum into hair follicles, which helps the hair from drying.

SUBCUTANEOUS LAYER

The subcutaneous layer is technically not skin, but rather anchors the skin to everything beneath. This layer provides support to the dermis and is comprised mainly of adipose tissue or fat. Some of us have more fat than others, but this layer is always present in some form. The fat store within this layer protects internal structures and insulates us against the cold (Timmons 2005), while the blood vessels in the subcutaneous layer feed and drain the capillaries of the dermis.

THE PHYSIOLOGY OF WOUND HEALING

The human body has an innate ability to repair damaged tissue (Russell 2002). When the skin is damaged, a sequence of processes occur which are interdependent, overlapping and aim to restore the normal structure and function of the skin (Dealey 2005). The repair is dependent on the type and depth of injury (Tortora and Grabowski 2003). The physiology of healing is complex and is often affected by a number of internal and external influences.

Wound healing can be divided into four dynamic phases.

1. Vascular response/Haemostasis (immediate response which can last up to five days)

The vascular response is not considered a stage in healing by some authors but has been included here to ensure that a full explanation of the body's response to skin damage is provided.

Following an injury, wounds can produce copious amounts of blood and serous fluid. Although bleeding has a cleansing effect on the wound in that surface contaminants are washed away (Dealey and Cameron 2008), the body responds by constricting the damaged blood vessels to minimise blood loss. This process is initiated by the injured blood vessel secreting a substance which initiates a process referred to as haemostasis. Haemostasis includes three major steps: (1) vasoconstriction (vessels shrink); (2) temporary blockage of a break in the vessel by a platelet plug; and (3) blood coagulation and formation of a clot to seal the hole until the tissue is repaired.

2. Inflammatory response (normal duration 3–7 days)

The inflammatory phase is the body's natural response to injury. Once haemostasis has been achieved, blood vessels dilate and their permeability increases to allow essential cells, antibodies, white blood cells, growth factors, enzymes and nutrients to reach the damaged area. This leads to a rise in exudate levels (fluid rich in white blood cells and platelets) and the skin may appear red and swollen and be painful due to injured nerves (Dealey 2005).

The white blood cells engulf and destroy bacteria and debris while growth factors stimulate the division of endothelial cells and direct the growth of new blood vessels (Tortora and Grabowski 2003). Waldrop and Doughty (2000) note that chronic wounds can become stuck in a vicious cycle in which a prolonged inflammatory phase serves to cause further tissue damage.

3. Proliferation (normal duration 3–25 days)

During this phase the wound is 'rebuilt' with new granulation tissue. Granulation tissue is the new wound matrix. It is made up of collagen and ground substance, has a granular appearance and is a pinky red colour. During this phase epithelial cells resurface the wound, in a process known as 'epithelialisation'. The wound contracts as epithelial cells and hair follicles increase in number and migrate across the wound bed. When the two migrating wound surfaces come together resurfacing is complete and 'contact inhibition' occurs (Timmons 2005). This stage of the healing process is dependent upon the cells receiving sufficient levels of oxygen and nutrients supplied by the blood vessels.

4. Maturation (normal duration 25 days to one year)

During this phase the tensile strength of the skin increases. Type III collagen laid down during the proliferation stage is gradually replaced with a stronger more defined collagen (Type I). This collagen is laid down in a more orderly network and the blood supply decreases, resulting in a smoother, flatter, paler scar. Mature scars are avascular and contain no hair, sebaceous or sweat glands.

CLASSIFICATIONS OF WOUNDS

Wounds are often categorised into acute or chronic, and heal by primary or secondary intention. There are principally two types of acute wound: traumatic wounds and surgical wounds. A traumatic wound includes minor cuts and abrasions through to extensive tissue injuries which are caused when a force exceeds the strength of the skin or the underlying supporting tissues. This would include breaks in the skin caused by a fall or incurred during a fight, while surgical wounds involve an incision in the skin which is usually carried out by a skilled surgeon but can also be the result of self-harm. Acute wounds breach the integrity of the skin but are commonly short in duration as the skin is normally healthy with no internal pathological cause of the injury.

If the edges of an acute wound are in close proximity, then it will heal via primary intention. Primary intention occurs when there is no tissue loss. As minimal new granulation tissue is required, the body can usually heal the breach in the skin without complications. Surgical tape, tissue adhesive, steri-strips, sutures or staples may be used to hold the wound margins together while this process takes place.

Chronic wounds differ significantly from acute wounds. They are often caused by an underlying pathology, such as vascular insufficiency, which produces repeated insults to the tissues and disrupts the healing process. In acute wounds, if all the healing factors are in place, the wound will heal with very little interference from the health care professional whereas chronic wounds are much more difficult to heal.

There are many definitions of chronic wounds. A wound is generally referred to as chronic when, despite appropriate treatment, it has shown no improvement for 2–3 months. However, this does not encompass the full range of wounds that are considered to be chronic, for example re-occurring wounds. Collier (2002) defined chronic wounds as those that are failing to heal as anticipated or that have become fixed at any one phase of wound healing. There are a wide range of chronic wounds, including leg ulcers, burns, diabetic ulcers and pressure ulcers, all of which may be encountered in mental health practice.

Chronic wounds heal by secondary intention, whereby the edges of the wound are left to close on their own. With chronic wounds there is usually a cavity or void and healing occurs through formation of large amounts of granulation tissue (Timmons 2005). The wound gradually contracts and epithelial cells migrate across the void to close the wound.

The process of wound healing and consequent wound management required will be determined in no small part by the type of wound the client has and whether healing will be by primary or secondary intention.

FACTORS WHICH IMPACT ON WOUND HEALING

Although the majority of wounds heal without incident, it is essential to have an understanding of the influence of the many interrelated factors which can affect these processes (Bale and Jones 2006) (see Table 9.3). Of particular relevance to this client group is the impact of diabetes on wound healing, given the prevalence of this disease among those with a mental health problem (see Chapter 3).

Before moving on, take some time to apply your understanding of wound healing by completing Action Learning Point 9.1.

Action Learning Point 9.1

Identify a client with a wound and consider the following:

- Is it an acute or chronic wound?
- Will it heal by primary or secondary intention?
- What phase of healing is it in?
- What factors may help and hinder the healing process in this case?

Table 9.3 Factors which affect wound healing

Intrinsic and extrinsic factors	Effect on wound healing
Psychological and physiological stress	Stress delays wound healing due to stimulation of the sympathetic nervous system as it causes vasoconstriction, reducing perfusion of the wound.
Diabetes	Compromised circulation in diabetic clients leads to a high risk of developing diabetic ulcers and significant delays in wound healing.
Lifestyle factors, including obesity and smoking	Smoking and obesity impact on circulation and result in a reduced amount of blood, oxygen and nutrients at the wound bed.
Age	All phases of wound healing are affected by aging slowing the process down.
Nutrition	Nutrition has a vital role to play in the process of wound healing (Perkins 2000). As a result of being deprived of one or more essential nutrients, some wounds may become 'stuck' at a certain stage during the wound healing process (Lansdown 2004).
Dehydration	Dehydration can have a negative effect on wound healing and fluid and nutritional loss may increase in patients who have heavily exuding wounds (Gunnewicht and Dunford 2004).
Corticosteroid medication	Raised levels of corticosteroids suppress the inflammatory and immune responses and hence delay wound healing and reduce resistance to infection.
Pressure	Compression of the tissue between bone and a hard surface restricts the blood supply to the skin, causing pressure sores to develop and any existing wounds in that area to be significantly compromised.
Shear and friction	Shearing or friction can remove any granulating tissue from the wound bed and delay healing.
Infection	The presence of a wound infection causes tissue damage and leads the wound to deteriorate.
Moisture	Moisture balance is vital to wound healing as excess moisture impedes healing, causing the breakdown of granulating tissue. Inadequate moisture in the wound environment, related primarily to exposure of the wound environment to air, dries the wound resulting in poorer wound healing rates.

THE ROLE OF THE MENTAL HEALTH PRACTITIONER

Effective wound care in mental health practice is dependent upon the practitioner's ability to assess, plan, implement and evaluate evidence-based wound care while affording consideration to the complex needs of each individual client. Indeed, if wound healing is to be maximised then it is paramount that any underlying diseases and health conditions are assessed and managed in addition to the wound.

WOUND ASSESSMENT

Accurate wound assessment is essential to the appropriate and realistic planning of goals and interventions for clients with wounds. However, Fettes (2006) notes that current methods of wound assessment are often subjective and inconsistent. Ideally, the process of assessment should be systematic and the content should include the following:

- The number and location of wounds.
- The size of the wound: the dimensions (length and breadth) can be measured using a plastic ruler (which should be disinfected) or approximated from a tracing on a proprietary measuring grid.
- The nature of any wound fluid: Cuzzell (1988) recommends describing the material in the wound simplistically using a colour classification as an adjunct to the descriptor:

    o yellow (sloughy) – slough; dead cells accumulated
    o black (necrotic) – dead tissue
    o green (infected) – pus with offensive odour; signs of inflammation
    o red (granulating) – granulating tissue
    o pink (epithelialising) – white/pink tissue

- The grade of the wound(s): a wide range of wound assessment tools are available for different types of wound (see Table 9.4 for an example).
- The cause, nature and severity of any pain related to the wound: this may be determined using a pain assessment scale.

Ideally, the continuity of the assessment process should be maintained with the same person reassessing the wound on each occasion to maximise the possibility that changes in its condition will be identified. Where this is not possible, detailed documentation should be maintained to record the assessment process and provide subsequent professionals with comprehensive information regarding the condition of the wound. Documentary evidence should detail whether the dressing therapy is effective in so far as it is managing the exudate effectively, controlling any odour, not the cause of discomfort or pain and is acceptable to the client. The ongoing assessment should

Table 9.4 Classification of pressure ulcers (European Pressure Ulcer Advisory Panel 2009)

Grade 1 – This stage is described as non-blanchable erythema of intact skin. This is detected by the blanching test: when a finger is gently pressed against healthy tissue that is lightly coloured, the skin blanches or turns white. If, on applied pressure, a questionable spot maintains its red, blue or purple hue and does not blanch, it is classed as a grade 1 pressure ulcer as this indicates damage to the dermal blood supply. Discolouration of the skin, warmth, oedema or hardness can also be used as indicators, particularly on individuals with darker skin.
Grade 2 – Partial thickness skin loss involving epidermis or dermis, or both. The ulcer is superficial and presents clinically as an abrasion or blister.
Grade 3 – Full thickness skin loss involving damage to or necrosis of subcutaneous tissue that may extend down to, but not through, underlying fascia.
Grade 4 – Extensive destruction, tissue necrosis or damage to muscle, bone or supporting structures with/without full thickness skin loss.

Source: European Pressure Ulcer Advisory Panel and National Pressure Ulcer Advisory Panel (2009) *Prevention and Treatment of Pressure Ulcers: Quick Reference Guide*. Washington, DC: National Pressure Ulcer Advisory Panel.

also consider changes in the size and shape of the wound, the odour produced, as well as the presence of any signs of inflammation and infection. The condition of the surrounding skin should also be examined to ensure that the wound exudates and/or the adhesive dressings are not causing damage to the skin surface.

It is vital that any wound assessment also includes the practitioner looking to identify any signs of infection. Although micro-organisms are present in all wounds, this does not indicate wound infection and accurately identifying the presence of an infection can be a challenge to health care professionals due to the subtle nature of some of the clinical indicators. The 'classic' signs of wound infection include changes to the visual appearance of the wound, such as localised redness and swelling or discoloration at the wound margins. The wound may also become increasingly pain-ful and feel hot, and the discharge may become viscous, resemble pus and have a purulent smell. Upon changing wound dressings it may be observed that the wound is friable and bleeds despite gentle handling. In addition, the presence of an infec-tion may lead to delayed healing and you may not encounter any other symptoms but find that the wound is failing to heal as anticipated or may even deteriorate and begin to break down (Cutting and Harding 1994).

It is also useful to remember that there are occasions when the signs of a wound infection may not be present but there are other changes to the client's general condition, such as an elevated temperature or general lethargy, which may indicate the presence of an infection (Collier 2004). A definitive diagnosis of infection is usually through clinical observation and judgement, and advice should be sought when confirmation of wound infection is required (European Wound Management Association 2006). Wound swabbing is the most frequently used sampling method and once infection has been confirmed and antibiotic sensitivities identified, appropriate treatment regimens can be implemented (Collier 2004). In the event that a wound becomes infected, systemic antibiotics are used but broad spectrum treatments are not advocated due to the emergence of resistant strains. Topical anti-microbials are also an alternative established treatment used for the management of infected wounds.

Pressure ulcers (PU) present a particular challenge to health care professionals as the underlying pathological causes are multifaceted. A PU is a localised injury to the skin and/or underlying tissue usually over a bony prominence, as a result of pressure or pressure in combination with shear. A number of contributing or confounding factors are also associated with pressure ulcers and the full significance of these factors is yet to be elucidated (European Pressure Ulcer Advisory Panel 2009). Direct pressure is the major causative factor in the development of PUs, and this occurs when the soft tissue of the body is compressed between a bony prominence and a hard surface which occludes the blood supply and leads to ischemia and tissue death (Wounds UK 2006).

A further causative factor is shear force, in which the skeleton and underlying tissue move down the bed or chair under gravity, while the skin on the buttocks and back remain stuck to the same point on the mattress or chair. Twisting and dragging also occlude the blood vessels and cause ischaemia, which usually leads to the development of more extensive tissue damage (Wounds UK 2006). Shear force can be further exacerbated by the presence of surface moisture through incontinence or sweating (Dealey 2005) and by friction when the skin slides over the surface with which it is in contact. Friction occurs when two surfaces move or rub across one another, for example when new shoes rub and cause a blister to the heel. If the pressure is unrelieved for a long period of time, the damage can extend all of the way through the tissue to the bone. Altering an individual's position, or nursing them on an appropriate support surface in conjunction with position changes, can prevent pressure damage (Wounds UK 2006).

Despite the presence of preventative measures many individuals do go on to develop pressure ulcers and effective assessment is paramount in ensuring that appropriate care is delivered. The assessment of pressure ulcers should include a determination as to the grade of the ulcer (see Table 9.4), which identifies the level of severity and will facilitate the practitioner in determining the subsequent treatment and management.

In the case of many elderly people with mental health problems their medication and/or the actual mental health condition itself, for example Parkinsonism, may lead to movement disorders, such as constant rocking, which have the potential to increase the shearing and friction forces on the pressure areas. Mental health practitioners are advised to engage in preventative risk management strategies. There are numerous pressure ulcer prevention risk assessment tools available and the choice of tool is dependent on clinical environment and appropriateness to practice (NICE 2005). In the event that a client does develop a PU, a full assessment should be conducted and pressure area care provided. The wound healing should be facilitated by appropriate cleansing and dressing procedures as per all chronic wounds. Dependent on the severity of pressure ulcer or risk to the service user, it may be necessary to obtain a specialised support surface through consultation with a specialist practitioner. Take a look at Action Learning Point 9.2.

Action Learning Point 9.2

Conduct a wound assessment and document your findings. Then ask one of your colleagues to read the information and provide you with feedback regarding any omissions.

WOUND MANAGEMENT

The overarching aims of wound management in the immediate term are to control any bleeding and remove any foreign bodies that could act as a focus for infection in the wound. In the longer term, devitalised tissue, thick slough and pus should be removed, and an optimum environment conducive to the healing process should be maintained. The practitioner will then be promoting the formation of new granulation tissue and epithelialisation while protecting the wound against further trauma and pathogenic micro-organisms (Morris 2006). The correct intervention can greatly affect the time it takes to heal the wound, the quality of life for the individual during this time and the resultant scar. With any wound, adequate pain control is essential as this will reduce anxiety and discomfort for the client. Analgesia should be administered in a timely fashion to optimise clients' comfort during dressing changes. However, for some service users with wounds, in palliative care for example, healing is not the ultimate aim, but rather a symptom management approach is adopted.

WOUND CLEANSING

Having conducted a thorough wound assessment, the mental health practitioner must consider the means of cleaning and dressing the wound. The evidence base regarding which cleaning solutions should be used is inconclusive (Angeras et al. 1992; Griffiths et al. 2001; Fernandez et al. 2002), with debate centring on the use of warmed tap water or sterile saline solutions. The advantages of water include a reduction in cost as well as ease of accessibility, particularly in community settings. However, water is hypotonic and if used incorrectly and too frequently can cause oedema as it is absorbed into the wound bed, increasing wound exudate (Cunliffe and Fawcett 2002). Sterile 0.9% saline is isotonic and is routinely used as a cleansing solution in hospital settings as it does not donate or draw fluid away from a wound (Blunt 2001). Isotonic solutions do not impede normal wound healing or damage tissue and, as such, saline is recommended as the cleaning fluid of choice. However, where this is not available there is evidence to suggest that warmed tap water can also be used without ill effect to the service user (Flanagan 1997). The way in which the wound is cleaned also has a significant effect on the healing process. Heavily exudating wounds may need to be cleaned by using sterile gauze soaked in saline to remove the exudate, while irrigation (using a syringe to gently trickle cleaning solution across the wound bed) may be more appropriate in the case of granulating wounds with less exudate. Practitioners should be aware that swabbing a granulating wound bed may have the effect of removing the new granulating tissue and disrupt the healing process.

DRESSING SELECTION

Chronic wounds, such as PUs, require careful dressing selection to provide the optimum healing environment as selecting the appropriate treatment and product is essential to determine the suitability for application to a particular type of wound. In a seminal piece of research, Winter (1962) demonstrated that moist conditions encouraged healing, prevented dehydration and promoted migration of epithelial cells. Therefore the process of selecting the optimum dressing must include some consideration as to the dressing's fluid and odour-absorbing characteristics, ability to conform to the shape of the body area, its handling, adhesive and antibacterial properties (Thomas 1997). Other factors which may also influence product selection include the ease of application and removal (including the production of pain and trauma to wound surface) and the recommended time between dressing changes (Thomas 1997). Prior to the application of any wound/dressing product, it is essential that the manufacturer's instructions be read carefully. Failure to do this may result in the dressing being ineffective or even detrimental to the healing process.

Clients with a wound dressing may encounter discomfort and their wounds will often become itchy as the nerve endings regrow. As a result they may be tempted to remove or disturb the bandages to access the wound. This presents an infection risk and has the potential to damage the healing tissue. As such, all clients should be educated regarding the importance of adhering to treatment regimes. There may be occasions when the client is unable to fully understand or retain the information and mental health professionals may wish to factor this into the dressing selection process, perhaps opting for an alternative which can be more securely adhered. Take a few minutes to think about the following case study.

Maureen

Maureen is 85 years old and has recently been referred to the dementia service by her doctor. Maureen lives with her sister since the death of her husband three years ago. Her family have noticed a deterioration in her cognitive function as she has become increasingly forgetful and unaware of her surroundings. She recently had a chest infection which resulted in a hospital admission and due to extended periods in bed her hip is blistered and weeping and her heels have become red and painful, although the skin is not broken. Maureen is not receiving any care from physical care providers and she can mobilise, but is reluctant to do so due to fatigue. She sleeps on a standard divan mattress at home which is 15 years old and sits in a recliner chair.

- What physical health assessment should be undertaken and why?
- What factors will you need to consider when selecting a method of cleaning and dressing Maureen's wounds?
- Consider how you can best promote Maureen's wound healing.

(Continued)

CASE STUDY

(Continued)

Answer guide:

1   Maureen requires an assessment of her skin. The European Pressure Ulcer Advisory Panel's (2009) pressure ulcer classification scale can be used to identify the grade of Maureen's ulcerated heels and hip. Maureen's heels should be assessed using the blanching test to identify the presence of a Grade 1 pressure ulcer. Maureen's hip is a Grade 2 pressure ulcer and will require a dressing. It is important that attention is afforded to Maureen's other pressure areas, such as her sacrum and elbows, to ensure that any further tissue damage is identified as early as possible. In addition, the MHP could assess Maureen for the presence of factors which are known to impact on wound healing, paying particular attention to those listed in Table 9.3.
2   Maureen's wound can be cleansed with saline, or tap water if that is not available. The wound on her hip is in a difficult place to dress and will require a highly flexible dressing which is able to conform to the shape of her body. Given that the wound is weeping, the dressing will also need to be highly absorbent and consideration must be afforded to the time needed between dressing changes.

The MHP should refer Maureen to the community nursing service to ensure that an appropriate package of care is put into place. Maureen and her sister could also be educated regarding the importance of mobilising and changing position regularly. In addition, they should ensure that Maureen is encouraged to maintain her hydration and stay well-nourished to promote effective wound healing. If necessary, Maureen should be discouraged from disturbing the dressing.

In contrast to chronic wounds such as PUs, self-inflicted wounds tend to be of a superficial and uncomplicated nature (NICE 2004b). As such, the treatment of the wound itself may well be relatively straightforward. However, given the aetiology of the wider condition, management may be much more complex.

NICE guidelines (2004b) indicate that in the UK the majority of wounds inflicted by self-cutting are less than 5 cm in length and are relatively easy to close. Akin to any other traumatic wounds, the initial management should involve emergency first aid procedures such as stemming the bleeding and assessing for the presence of foreign bodies, abraded or loose skin and infection (Benbow and Deacon 2011), before covering the wound with an appropriate dressing such as a tissue adhesives and skin closure strips if required.

NICE guidelines (2004b) emphasise the need for the service user to be involved in any treatment decisions, which should take account of the client's preferred treatment method, including the facilitation of self-care. Taylor et al. (2009) believe that self-care should be placed within a positive and respectful therapeutic relationship and as part of this practitioners may wish to provide their clients with advice and direction regarding self-management. The following guidance, offered by Benbow and Deacon (2011: 31), may thus prove valuable to both mental health practitioners and their clients.

1   Ensure that a first-aid kit is accessible and ready for use.
2   After self-wounding, stay calm, breathe slowly and reassure yourself that you are going to look after yourself as well as possible.
3   Ensure that your hands are clean and dry.
4   Stem bleeding by applying gentle pressure to wounds with a clean cloth that will not disintegrate and leave debris in the wound.
5   Clean the wound with warmed bottled or drinkable tap water. Cuts benefit from large volumes of fluid applied at constant high pressure from a tap.
6   When the bleeding has stopped and the wound has been cleaned, make sure the edges are dry.
7   Close the wound using tissue adhesive or surgical tape.

Returning to the complexity of this issue, we acknowledge that this chapter has focused largely on the wound care needs of service users who self-harm, which will form only a small part of the wider package of care required by this client group. We therefore refer the reader to Ousey and Ousey (2010), who emphasise the need for individuals who self-harm to have a full mental health and social needs assessment and ask that such an assessment includes the identification of the specific motivational factors which influence the individual to self-injure.

CONCLUSION

Service users in mental health are susceptible to both acute and chronic wounds and health care professionals working in the field have an important role to play in ensuring these individuals receive the correct treatment and management. This necessitates an understanding of wound healing processes, an ability to conduct a thorough systematic wound assessment, and the provision of optimal wound care. Engaging the service user in the management of their wounds can, where appropriate, be a preferable and empowering experience, while utilising a holistic assessment and care package can ensure that the specific, and perhaps wider, needs of each individual client are considered and addressed.

USEFUL RESOURCES

At the time of writing in the UK we recommend the following resources:

MIND (self-harm) – www.mind.org.uk/help/diagnoses_and_conditions/self-harm
Royal College of Psychiatrists – www.rcpsych.ac.uk/mentalhealthinfoforall/problems/depression/self-harm.aspx
European Wound Management Organisation – http://ewma.org/
Worldwide Wounds – www.worldwidewounds.com/

10

PRESCRIBING IN MENTAL HEALTH PRACTICE – THE BALANCING ACT

BEN GREEN

Learning outcomes:

By the end of this chapter you should be able to:

- Discuss the potential impact of psychiatric pharmacology on the physical health of individuals with mental health problems
- Consider the potential impact of medical prescribing on the mental health of such individuals
- Reflect on the role of the mental health practitioner in medication management

---

INTRODUCTION

Psychiatric prescribing undoubtedly has a major role in the treatment of mental health conditions, alleviating symptoms, assisting recovery and enabling people with such conditions to gain the stability they need for rehabilitation and psycho-therapy. Nevertheless, such prescribing benefits can also incur a cost in terms of adverse effects, from drowsiness to coronary heart disease. This chapter addresses the effects on physical health caused by the prescription of psychiatric drugs and, conversely, mental health problems associated with medical prescribing. Some of the main physical problems associated with psychiatric prescribing will also be considered, including side-effects, drug safety and drug–drug interactions. The chapter finally discusses the means by which psychiatric prescribing can best be monitored and managed more safely.

Epidemiological studies repeatedly show that most people with mental health problems are not diagnosed and are not treated (by counselling, psychotherapies or prescribed drugs). Even so, the scale of prescribing of psychiatric drugs is huge and increasing, with primary care physicians calling on their use in about 50% of the cases of mental health problems they identify (Linden et al. 1999).

Some countries have tried to address this by using psychological therapies as first-line options for anxiety and depression and yet the trend for prescribing persists. Outside any discussion of the relative therapeutic values of the various treatment options, it is prudent to note that roughly 10% of all health service expenditure, in the UK, is on medicines and the cost of prescribing rose more than tenfold between 1980 and 2007 (Office of Health Economics 2009). The huge scope of psychiatric prescribing is worth considering for various reasons, but key to this chapter is the fact that there are many physical implications of these medicines and with their increased use such implications are becoming more prevalent.

PSYCHIATRIC PRESCRIBING FOR INDIVIDUALS WITH MENTAL HEALTH PROBLEMS

THE DRUGS DO WORK!

Before embarking on what will be a dauntingly long list of the negative aspects of psychiatric prescribing, it is worth considering briefly whether the positive aspects outweigh the negative. In short, do the benefits outweigh the risks? On balance, I believe the benefits far outweigh the risks, but there will be counter-arguments, sometimes forceful and well-reasoned. Other counter-arguments are sometimes philosophical or perhaps overly optimistic regarding the severe and pervasive nature of mental illness.

One way to consider the impact of the twentieth-century advances in psychiatric pharmacology is to reflect on the consequences of severe mental illness (SMI) prior to the introduction of first-generation antipsychotic medication in the 1950s. During this time the long-term nature of SMI, together with the relatively low frequency of spontaneous recovery, led to a progressive accumulation of patients in asylums. In 1870 there were 27,109 psychiatric beds in England and Wales. In 1910 there were 97,580 (Gregory 2004). At the start of the National Health Service (NHS) in 1948 over half of all NHS beds were psychiatric beds (Figure 10.1). However, something happened to reverse this expansion. The bed numbers peaked at 148,100 in 1954 (Gregory 2004). Thereafter there was a rapid and persistent decline in bed numbers so that in 2007 (when the UK population was 60,943,912), there were only 20,000 or so psychiatric beds. This is a similar number to the late 1800s when the population was about 17 million or a third of that in 2007 (Green 2009).

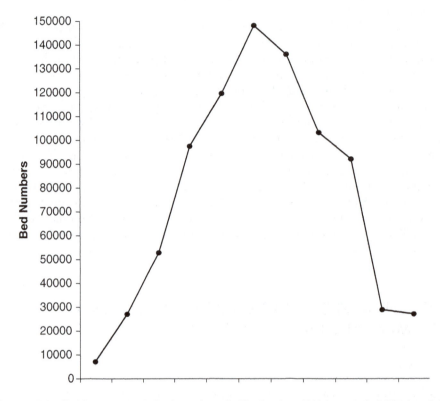

Figure 10.1   Public psychiatric bed numbers in England and Wales 1850–2007 (peak in 1954) (Green 2009)

The fall in psychiatric bed occupancy starting in the 1950s pre-dates any political move towards community care and is based upon the efficacy of a new class of drugs (the dopamine blockers), antipsychotics such as chlorpromazine (first synthesised in 1950 and first used in psychiatry in 1952) and others such as haloperidol (1958) and levomepromazine (1959) (Green 2004).

It was the success of these drugs which enabled patients to be discharged from the psychiatric hospitals back into the community. Sometimes the effects were remarkably quick. Hospital records from this time include case histories where patients admitted for decades were able to be discharged after weeks on the new drugs.

The argument can thus be made for the dramatic efficacy of psychiatric medication in the treatment of mental illness. For the first time in millennia, humankind has had the means to treat mental illness and alleviate suffering, preventing the need for the incarceration of the majority of mentally ill people. Without the use of such drugs we arguably might require an asylum-building programme of unthinkable proportions.

Having made the public health case for psychiatric medication, we must now turn to the individual's experiences of such drugs, which are not always completely positive. It can be argued that some adverse physical effects are infinitely preferable to decades of in-patient care for schizophrenia, or years of severe depression, but to inform such an argument we must first increase our awareness of the extent of the physical effects of some medications.

WHAT IS THE COST TO PHYSICAL HEALTH?

All medicines are associated with side-effects or adverse effects. These are difficult to classify. Some of the effects are predictable, based upon the drug's known pharmacology, and others are somewhat unpredictable or idiosyncratic. Those working in mental health care should consider the relative advantages of medication as well as the prevalence and severity of any negative side-effects. Unfortunately, psychiatric medication exposes individuals with a mental health problem to a wide a range of serious physical health conditions, such as diabetes (see Chapter 3) and cardiovascular problems (see Chapter 4), while also causing physical adverse effects which can impact on the individual's daily functioning. A drug like chlorpromazine, for instance, is thought to derive its main antipsychotic effects from blocking dopamine receptors in the brain (D_2 receptors), but it also affects other receptors, such as histamine. Its effects on histamine receptors cause the drowsiness associated with the drug. In one way the sedation is an unwanted or adverse effect. In another sense, for overactive and disturbed patients with insomnia this side-effect becomes a desired effect. We can also predict its Parkinsonian-like side-effects (tremor and muscle rigidity) from its effects on cholinergic receptors, and its tendency to cause postural hypotension on its effects on adrenergic receptors. Its more unpredictable or idiosyncratic effects are less easy to predict from pharmacology and are derived from experience with the drug over many years – such as the photosensitive skin suffered by people who take chlorpromazine (and a consequent need for topical sun-blocking agents).

One of the key problems faced by individuals with mental health problems when taking medicines is that their complaints about them are often attributed to their underlying illness. No one can know every side-effect of a drug and even the literature does not always record them all. This can lead to problems when the health professional discounts the individual's experience. I shudder with embarrassment and hesitate to disclose that as a student I found it difficult to credit a young woman's account of lactation on an antipsychotic and a male patient's complaint that on an antipsychotic he was 'firing blanks' when he masturbated. A little more experience talking to clients and reading about psychopharmacology taught me the error of my ways! New drugs are also sometimes marketed without all the side-effects being known. Again, listening to the client is key. Shortly after paroxetine was marketed in the 1990s I noted that it was a very good antidepressant and very good at allaying anxiety, but I also had clients telling me, after some time on the drug, that they felt very tearful if they failed to take the medication for a few days. Some described towering rages; others described 'electric zap sensations' or 'a series of images over-lapping when I turn my head'. You can see how easy it might be to assume these were symptoms of illness. The pharmaceutical company was not much help in iden-tifying these experiences. It was only when dozens of clients described these symp-toms and doctors started talking together about them that the unusual descriptions gathered value as descriptions of withdrawal effects.

THE PHYSICAL IMPACT OF PSYCHIATRIC MEDICATION

The relationship between physical and mental health is complex and psychiatric medication has been implicated as a causative factor in a wide range of adverse physical effects and conditions.

WEIGHT GAIN

While effective against psychosis, many of our current antipsychotic drugs promote weight gain, and in such clients there appears to be a higher incidence of weight-related disorders such as diabetes and coronary heart disease. In particular, second-generation antipsychotic medication, once enthusiastically endorsed by pharmaceutical companies and agencies such as the National Institute for Health and Clinical Excellence (NICE), have now been found to promote weight gain, especially clozapine and olanzapine (Tschoner et al. 2009). For example, the body mass increase with these can be a significant (25% +) long-term increase. Over 10 weeks' treatment with clozapine, Allison et al. (2009) found that the average service user put on 4.45 kg; with olan-zapine this was 4.15kg; and with risperidone it was 2.15 kg.

Weight gain is not confined to antipsychotics. Many antidepressants, if used long term, also stimulate weight gain and this too is associated with the development of metabolic syndrome (Andersohn et al. 2009). Implicated antidepressants include amitriptyline, paroxetine and mirtazapine.

Apart from the physical risks associated with these complications, patients do not like an altered appearance, as can be seen in Hamer and Haddad's (2007) study where 73% of patients reported concern about weight gain. This was particularly prevalent in women and a consequent effect on compliance was noted.

In view of these problems, guidelines now state the need for prescribers to con-sider physical health factors such as diabetes, or family history of diabetes, and conduct relevant tests before embarking on antipsychotic therapy. A cautionary note should be sounded about the use of antipsychotic drugs outside their intended field. Sometimes, because of the side-effect of sedation, antipsychotics can be used as sleeping tablets or as anxiolytics. This kind of use can be legitimate, but it is also off licence – that is, neither the pharmaceutical company nor the state regulatory bodies would readily sanction the use of the drug for off licence uses. This leaves the client in a position of being able, in the event of an adverse reaction, to recover damages from the prescriber only, rather than from the usually wealthier pharmaceutical company. For instance, a prescriber could find themselves sued for prescribing olanzapine to a client with anxiety disorder who later developed diabetes, especially without ensuring the client had been through the necessary screening for diabetes risks beforehand.

There are many ways of minimising weight gain and some of the key considerations are outlined below:

- Consider antipsychotics that are least associated with weight gain, particularly in clients with a family history of cardiac problems and/or diabetes
- Recent research has noted the possibility of using metformin in treating olanzapine-induced weight gain (Praharaj 2011), although switching antipsychotics would seem more practical than exposing a client to two drugs where a single alternative might do
- Dietary education/modification, for example healthy eating programmes
- Exercise programmes, coaching and training, such as referral on prescription schemes
- Weight monitoring programmes, examples of which can be found in Chapter 11

METABOLIC SYNDROME AND DIABETES

The link between a metabolic syndrome of obesity and insulin resistance and schizophreniform illness has been appreciated for some time. In 1897 Henry Maudsley (of the Maudsley Hospital, London) noted 'diabetes is a disease which often shows itself in families where insanity prevails' (Green 2009). This basic link between schizophrenia and a metabolic syndrome is explored in Chapter 3 but its relevance to this particular chapter is in the fact that antipsychotic drugs often increase weight, as outlined above, which consequently increases not only the risk of metabolic syndrome and diabetes but also that of cardiovascular diseases (Allison et al. 2009).

CARDIOVASCULAR DISEASES

For individuals with mental health problems the risk of developing cardiovascular disease is two to three times greater than that of the general population, depending on where in the world the person lives (Hennekens et al. 2005; Filik et al. 2006). Part of the reason for this increased risk is again the increase in weight as a result of some of the medications, but it is also wider than this. Chapter 4 investigates cardiovascular disease in more detail but it is worth considering here the risk of postural hypotension, which can be a side-effect of some antidepressants and antipsychotics. It is related to alpha-1 blockade, which is produced by drugs like chlorpromazine, amitriptyline, venlafaxine and others.

Postural hypotension (or orthostatic hypotension) involves a drop of 10–20 mmHg in systolic blood pressure on changing of posture from sitting to standing, which may lead to dizziness, fainting sensations and falls (and thus to hip fractures in the elderly).

The management of postural hypotension includes monitoring the service user's blood pressure on a regular basis. Being alert to complaints of dizziness is also important, as is acting on these by checking blood pressure both while the client is sitting and standing.

If postural hypotension is present, consider using an alternative drug – especially in older patients who might fall. Until the old drug is replaced, give a full explanation about the risks of sudden movements to both the client and their family/carers, and advise them about standing up gradually, and avoiding triggers such as high temperature environments, heavy meals and prolonged periods of standing still.

Also worthy of discussion is adult sudden death syndrome, which some clients may be exposed to due to the impact of psychiatric medication on the cardiovascular system. This is linked with drugs that can delay the repolarisation of heart muscle – measured on ECG by a QTc prolongation beyond 420 ms. This is seen in all antipsychotics, although Glassman and Bigger (2001) report that with first-generation antipsychotics the risk of sudden death syndrome is almost three times greater, although this is still very rare. Various risk factors are associated with sudden death syndrome and antipsychotics, including organic psychiatric disorder, hypertension, high body mass index, smoking and history of a myocardial infarction. Particularly risky antipsychotics for prolonging QTc on ECG are thioridazine and haloperidol. Various medical drugs are also associated with sudden death syndrome, including amiodarone (ironically this is an anti-arrhythmic).

An effective means of managing the risk of adult sudden death syndrome is tackling associated risks such as hypertension, weight reduction and smoking cessation in combination with informed prescribing. As a guideline, prescribers are advised to use low-risk drugs at the lowest effective dose. Monitoring baseline and regular ECGs looking for QTc prolongation will also facilitate early detection and treatment. Before moving on, take this opportunity to consider Action Learning Point 10.1.

Action Learning Point 10.1

- Discuss with your team how they routinely monitor ECG changes in clients on antipsychotics.

CANCER

There is a small body of literature which considers the possibility of a carcinogenic risk associated with psychiatric medication. In the USA, the Food and Drug Administration (FDA) requires extensive animal testing to determine the carcinogenic potential of drugs. For instance, drug information in the USA refers to the potential of, say, a very high dose of risperidone to induce pituitary adenomas in mice. The relevance to humans is not clearly established. Such tumours are thought to be related to prolonged dopamine D_2 antagonism and hyperprolactinaemia.

Hyperprolactinaemia occurs in about 40% of women on antipsychotics (excluding clozapine) (Bushe et al. 2008). It is probable that this area of research will grow in future years.

There is concern that some antipsychotic drugs can interfere with chemotherapy regimes. For instance, chemotherapy can affect the bone marrow and so can clozapine. Opinion is somewhat divided on whether clozapine therapy should be suspended during chemotherapy, but the limited evidence suggests continuation is not problematic (Goulet and Grignon 2008). Research is ongoing, however. See Chapter 6 for further information relating to the management of cancer.

SEXUAL SIDE-EFFECTS

Chapter 8 explores the sexual health of individuals with mental health problems. Here consideration will be given specifically to the effects of medication on sexual functioning.

Sexual side-effects (SSEs) of medication affect a person's quality of life and lead to poor compliance. Sexual side-effects may be experienced by about 43% of clients on antipsychotics (Wallace 2001). SSEs with antipsychotics can include loss of libido due to hyperprolactinaemia, erectile failures (e.g. 40% of men had difficulty in achieving and maintaining erection with chlorpromazine) and ejaculatory failures (e.g. total inhibition of ejaculation or even retrograde ejaculation) and priapism (painful prolonged erection of the penis or clitoris).

Selective serotonin reuptake inhibitors (SSRI) antidepressants can delay ejaculation in males so fluoxetine is sometimes used for treating premature ejaculation. The side-effect of delayed ejaculation/climax in males can be unpleasant for some couples and welcomed by others. The antidepressant clomipramine has been linked to complete anorgasmia. Clients frequently discontinue medication as a result of SSEs, which highlights the need for mental health practitioners to incorporate sexual health into their assessment and care. Unfortunately the research evidence indicates that professionals generally fail to even ask about SSEs. Most psychiatrists (77%) surveyed in a recent study, for instance, only explored the topic of SSEs when they were cued by clients (Singh et al. 2010). Sexual function can, of course, be compromised by psychiatric illness itself and by physical illness.

BLOOD DYSCRASIA

Blood dyscrasia is an abnormality of the blood and generally implies some disorder in the production of blood cell components, for instance insufficient erythrocytes (anaemia) or insufficient platelets (thrombocytopenia).

Clozapine, used in treatment resistant schizophrenia, can affect bone marrow function leading to reduced white cell production or even agranulocytosis (a more profound reduction of white cells which can become permanent). At the start of clozapine therapy, blood counts should therefore be monitored weekly.

Other drugs, like carbamazepine, chlorpromazine and zuclopenthixol, can also impair white cell production and mental health practitioners should be alert for the signs of infection in any client prescribed these drugs. They should also ensure that a white cell blood count is carried out in the event that they do develop an infection.

HYPERPROLACTINAEMIA

Prolactin is a hormone secreted by the pituitary gland. Various drugs, including antipsychotics, can trigger higher blood prolactin levels. Dopamine blockade by some antipsychotics leads to more prolactin. High levels of prolactin can cause infertility in women, through disturbance of, or absence of, the normal menstrual cycle. Hyperprolactinaemia can lead to lactation, amenorrhoea, gynaecomastia, vaginal dryness and hirsutism. Hyperprolactinaemia also occurs in men taking anti-psychotics and may lead to loss of libido or erectile dysfunction. Of all the antipsy-chotics, quetiapine is probably least likely to cause this side-effect.

A recent study found hyperprolactinaemia in a third of patients on antipsychotics, mainly in females (47.3% and 17.6% in males) and was associated with all antip-sychotics except clozapine (Bushe et al. 2008). The highest prevalence rates were found with amisulpride and risperidone. Long-term hyperprolactinaemia has been linked to osteoporosis, bone fractures, pituitary tumours and breast cancer (Bushe et al. 2008). An awareness of these side-effects should enable those engaged in the care of individuals with a mental illness to seek early treatment for their clients. In addition, consideration should be given to reducing the dose of the medication and also to switching it to a prolactin sparing antipsychotic. Now take a look at Action Learning Point 10.2.

Action Learning Point 10.2

- Discuss with your team what efforts they make to routinely detect hyperprolactinaemia.
- What measures do they take to tackle the long-term consequences of hyper-prolactinaemia?

MOVEMENT DISORDERS

Among the most common side-effects of psychiatric medication is a change to the client's gait, posture and movement. These are frequently distressing to clients, are stigmatising and target them for unwanted attention by others. Extrapyramidal symptoms (EPSES) are motor side-effects usually caused by antipsychotics acting on the dopamine system. They include drug-induced Parkinsonism, a dopamine-blockade-related side-effect which can include limb and hand tremor, abnormal gait, 'cog-wheel' or ratchet-like muscle tone, and mask-like faces – relieved by oral procyclidine or an equivalent. In addition, an unpleasant inner restlessness called akathisa can be observed by the client's abnormal walking or pacing about or fidgeting when seated. This inner agitation is so upsetting it can lead to thoughts of suicide or violence.

Dystonia can present as a sudden (acute dystonia) or late (tardive dystonia) persistent muscle contraction or spasm. The dystonia is often seen with first-generation antipsychotics like haloperidol (dystonia is also seen with the anti-emetic drug metoclopramide – Maxolon). Such dystonias are usually seen in the neck (30%), tongue (17%), jaw (15%), or as an oculogyric crisis (in which the eyes roll back, and neck arches) 6%, and as opisthotonus (body arching) in 3.5% (Swett 1975). Acute dystonia is involuntary and very frightening for the client. The management is by administration of procyclidine, which may need to be repeated. The drug that precipitated the dystonia should be avoided thereafter.

Finally, tardive dyskinesia occurs in 5–30% of patients treated with long-term first-generation antipsychotics (Kane et al. 1988) and involves repetitive, involuntary movements without purpose. These may consist of any of the following: movement of the lips and tongue, such as grimacing, lip smacking, lip pursing, sticking out of the tongue; rapid blinking; 'fluttering' of the fingers; rapid movements of the arms; truncal movements – twisting of the trunk of the body; toe tapping; and moving the leg up and down. Some historical descriptions of these kinds of movements in clients with schizophrenia pre-date the development of antipsychotics, so there is debate as to whether they are side-effects of medication or something to do with the central nervous system disease that is schizophrenia. Also tardive dyskinesia has been found in up to 14% of first-degree relatives of people with schizophrenia – that is to say, tardive dyskinesia is found in relatives who have never had antipsychotics (McCreadie et al. 2003).

Agencies like NICE initially recommended switching patients to new antipsychotics to avoid tardive dyskinesia. However, subsequent experience with the drugs has shown that second-generation antipsychotics are also associated with tardive dyskinesia. The clinical antipsychotic trials of intervention effectiveness (CATIE trial), for instance, found that 4.5% of patients on quetiapine and 2.2% of patients on risperidone developed tardive dyskinesia (Miller et al. 2008).

Abnormal movements can be measured and monitored using instruments like the Abnormal Involuntary Movement Scale (AIMS) (Munetz and Benjamin 1988) and Extrapyramidal Symptom Rating Scale (ESRS) (Simpson and Angus 1970).

Catatonia is a profound generalised condition where patients may hold rigid poses for hours and will seemingly be oblivious to any external stimuli. It has been described since the 1870s and although it may be classified as a reaction to medication by some, it is still of uncertain aetiology. It can be treated with hydration, benzodiazepines and electroconvulsive therapy (ECT).

Neuroleptic malignant syndrome (NMS) is an idiosyncratic reaction to a variety of medications, including antipsychotics, antidepressants and lithium. It occurs in about 0.5% of those taking antipsychotics (Adnet et al. 2000). Its aetiology is somewhat uncertain and may be a variant of a condition described many years ago called lethal catatonia. NMS is traditionally held to be a reaction to medication. It is associated with raised temperature, increased muscle tone, delirium and autonomic instability. It is associated with raised creatine phosphokinase blood levels. It has a mortality of about 10–15% and is a medical emergency (Adnet et al. 2000). In the event of NMS, medical help should be sought immediately. Medication should be stopped and on later re-introduction the client must be monitored very closely.

SEDATION

Psychiatric drugs which affect histaminergic neuroreceptors, like tricyclic anti-depressants and some antipsychotics, can be sedating. This is useful in control-ling behavioural disturbance and also in tackling insomnia. Sedation is also seen to a lesser or greater extent with many other psychiatric drugs, including the newer antidepressant and antipsychotics. Such sedation affects vigilance and the ability to respond quickly and appropriately when using machinery or driving and so clients need warning about this problem. Reassurance should, however, be given that sedation is often at its worst in the first couple of weeks and that after this point many people will develop a tolerance and the sedative effects will become less. Where sedation persists, the possibility of reducing the dose should be considered along with the potential for splitting the dose between morning and evening. Thought should also be given to the need for the sedative effect as switching to a less sedative drug may be an option. Please refer to Action Learn-ing Point 10.4

Action Learning Point 10.4

- Look up the side-effects of the psychiatric medication for one of your clients. What physical health conditions are they at potential risk of and how is this being managed?

THE ROLE OF THE MENTAL HEALTH PRACTITIONER

MINIMISING THE COST THROUGH EFFECTIVE MEDICATION MANAGEMENT

Despite the potential controversy surrounding psychiatric medication, it is still widely regarded as one of the major therapeutic tools available to mental health professionals. Unfortunately, the lack of service users' adherence to medication is a long-standing and global concern (World Health Organization 2003), and how best to encourage engagement in such an approach has therefore drawn wide interest. Two of the main influences on non-adherence are proposed to be adverse side-effects and a lack of collaborative care, which has led to the suggestion that any attempts to enhance adherence should include strategies aimed at minimising adverse effects and maximising service user involvement (World Health Organization 2003).

Concordance is the term used to describe these combined aims, and is an approach that recognises the adverse effects of medication – regarding non-adherence as a legitimate and understandable response from the service user. The MHP's role in such circumstances is to discuss the reasons for non-adherence with the service user and in doing so take the opportunity to assess for the presence of adverse effects.

Medication assessments can be undertaken at many points throughout the care process but it is useful at the initial assessment to take some historical information about previous experiences of medication in order to identify any potential physical effects. Asking directly about the physical health of the individual's family could also identify a predisposition to some of the physical conditions associated with psychiatric medication. This can then be factored into any treatment decisions made. The use of standardised and validated assessment tools is also advocated as an additional tool for assessment, with the intention of reducing the MHPs reliance on the service users' self-report and introducing a more objective measure (Jones and Jones 2005). There are many available but a commonly adopted tool is the Liverpool University Neuroleptic Rating Scale (LUNSERS) (Day et al. 1995) and the recommendation is to continue to use these tools to monitor changes throughout treatment. If you are working in a rehabilitation service or depot service, then you can use one of these with service users every 3–6 months to monitor for the presence of the adverse effects outlined. This would be a prompt to monitor ECG changes, the development of abnormal involuntary movements (AIMs), and so on. For suggestions on what to include if devising a tool for your own service, see Box 10.1.

Box 10.1   Suggestions for Devising an Assessment Tool

Suggested headings would be:

Weight, BMI, waist circumference, blood pressure, heart rate and rhythm, temperature, anticholinergic side-effects, EPSEs, AIMs, excess sedation, prolactin levels, creatine kinase levels, sexual function, diabetes symptoms, glucose levels, HBA1 levels, liver function tests, lipid levels, ECG, full blood count.

There are general best practice principles to follow when it comes to medication management, many of which have already been adopted in the previous discussions on minimising adverse effects. However, the following guidance focuses particularly on the collaborative nature of the process and starts with an open, honest discussion about the medication that has been prescribed, including both the beneficial effects and the potential negatives associated with that particular medication. It is the latter that MHPs tend to shy away from, which is understandable given that this information may prevent an individual from taking a potentially very beneficial medication. However, it is actually the lack of preparation for these negative effects that is of most concern to service users, thus ensuring that it is paramount to give sufficient information (Gray et al. 2005).

Asking service users what knowledge they already have of the medication can be a good opening to the discussion and can also be a good way of identifying any misconceptions or lack of understanding. These can then be used as the basis for introducing education around the signs and symptoms of the potential adverse effects, and it is worth considering providing the information in written form so that it can be taken away and referred back to at a later date. Both service users and their family and carers should be involved in these discussions, and all involved in the care should be encouraged to take a proactive approach in the monitoring and reporting of any such symptoms. Monitoring is also a key role for the MHP, who should be aware of the medication regimes of individual service users in order to check for any signs and symptoms of adverse effects.

Should any adverse effects become apparent, the care of the individual should be reviewed. It is recommended that thought be given to the medication and whether any changes to this would be beneficial and possible (as outlined under the different adverse effects) and also that lifestyle changes are considered. The provision of health promotion advice in relation to lifestyle choices and changes is a developing role for MHPs and more guidance on this can be found in Chapter 11. However, it is worth reinforcing at this point that the provision of such advice can be empowering for service users as it allows them to collaborate fully in their care and affords them the opportunity to take some control over their own health and wellbeing. Take a look at the case study of Sinita below for an example of medication management in practice.

CASE STUDY

Sinita

Sinita, aged 45, has a history of recurrent depression and was admitted to hospital in a very agitated state. While there it was decided that her antidepressant would be changed to amitriptyline, as all previous antidepressants had failed to provide lasting improvement. Sinita, however, was reluctant to comply and it was only when asked about this that the MHP was able to identify that Sinita thought that the medication would make her 'like a zombie'. It seems that others on the ward had told her that the heavy sedative effects would render her unable to do or feel anything and this had understandably made her hesitant. The MHP took the opportunity to inform Sinita about the potential side-effects of the medication, honestly acknowledging the sedative effect but pointing out that this would assist with her feelings of agitation. The other potential side-effects were then discussed (principally weight gain and metabolic syndrome) and Sinita was informed that there were ways in which these could be managed. The benefits of the medication were finally reinforced before a summary of the information was written down and given to Sinita.

The following day the MHP met with Sinita and her family to further discuss the medication and an agreement was made that she would take this if she and her family could be involved in the monitoring and management of the adverse effects. Further meetings were therefore arranged to facilitate more education around the signs and symptoms of potential effects and to discuss potential lifestyle changes.

AWARENESS OF INTERACTIONS WITH OTHER DRUGS

The greater the number of medications a client is taking the higher is the risk of a serious drug interaction and MHPs are advised to have an awareness of the potential for this. Many individuals with mental health problems will be prescribed psychiatric medication which may increase their risk of physical health problems, leading to further prescribed medications. Should these medications cause side-effects, yet more medication may be used in an attempt to address them and the outcome may well be polypharmacy and a significantly increased risk of drug interactions.

Interactions can arise where there is competition for the bodily systems that eliminate drugs from the body. For instance, most drugs are metabolised by the liver. Therefore clients taking multiple medications may be putting their liver under considerable strain. Furthermore, some drugs, such as carbamazepine, may increase the rate at which the liver metabolises other medications. This has the potential to lower the serum levels of these other drugs and lead to breakthrough symptoms such as psychosis or depression. Service users prescribed medicines that can affect liver function should be monitored for changes in their Liver Function Tests (LFTs).

A section at the back of the British National Formulary (BNF) (2010: Appendix 1) details the most important known interactions between various drugs. The section in the September 2010 BNF is closely printed and nearly 90 pages long, indicating the complexity and number of potential interactions. It is therefore impossible to summarise them all and each service user has to be thought about individually in terms of their age, sex, weight, physical state of health and other medications. Table 10.1 lists some examples of interactions. Before moving on, think about Action Learning Point 10.5.

Action Learning Point 10.5

- Audit the number of prescribed drugs that each of the clients in your care is on. What is the mean number of medications? Could this be safely reduced? If so how?
- What would be the potential risks and benefits of reducing the number of medications for each client?

Table 10.1 Common drug–drug interactions

Physical health medication	Mental health medication	Effects of interaction
Ibuprofen, aspirin and other non-steroidal anti-inflammatory drugs	Lithium SSRI antidepressants and venlafaxine	Lithium toxicity Increased risk of bleeding

(Continued)

Table 10.1   (Continued)

Physical health medication	Mental health medication	Effects of interaction
ACE inhibitors (used in hypertension)	Antipsychotics, beta-blockers and MAOIs	Hypotension
Amiodarone (anti-arrhythmic)	Lithium, amisulpride and other antipsychotics	Arrhythmias
Anticonvulsants	SSRIs, tricyclics, carbamazepine, haloperidol, olanzapine, quetiapine, risperidone, Fluoxetine, mirtazapine, paroxetine	Lower fit threshold Impact on the concentration of psychiatric and/or anticonvulsant medication
Anaesthetics	Tricyclic antidepressants	Arrythmia and hypotension
Diuretics (used to treat heart failure, liver cirrhosis, hypertension and certain kidney diseases)	Tricyclics	Hypotension
	Lithium	Increased risk of lithium toxicity
Oestrogens (in oral contraceptives and HRT)	Tricyclics	Impair antidepressant effect
	Lamotrigine	Reduce serum levels of lamotrigine
Thyroid hormones	Antidepressants	Enhanced effect
Antifungals	Aripiprazole, quetiapine alprazolam and midazolam	Increases concentration of psychiatric medication
	Pimozide	Arrthymias
Histamine antagonists (used for oesophageal reflux)	Citalopram, mirtazapine, imipramine, chlorpromazine and benzodiazepines	Increases concentration of psychiatric medication
Methyldopa (antihypertensive)	MAOIs, anxiolytics and hypnotics.	Hypotension
Metoclopramide (anti-emetic)	Antipsychotics	Increased risk of Extrapyramidal Side Effects

AWARENESS OF THE PSYCHOLOGICAL EFFECTS OF PHYSICAL HEALTH MEDICATION

Given the propensity for physical illness in individuals with mental health problems, a further area of consideration for MHPs is the psychological effects of physical health medication. Several of these medications can cause symptoms of depression, anxiety and even psychosis and in such instances it is not uncommon for individuals to acquire new diagnoses or extra treatments they do not need. It is therefore important that MHPs are alert to the possibility that new psychological symptoms, or a worsening of existing symptoms, may be a result of medication that has been prescribed for the service user's physical health and that they liaise with the care team if they suspect that medical prescribing is having a psychological effect. Table 10.2 identifies a range of physical health medication and the potential psychological side-effects and Harry's case illustrates how such effects may present in practice.

Harry

Harry, a 72 year-old man, was under the care of the mental health team for long-standing moderate anxiety. Over the past two months it had been noted that his anxiety had become significantly worse and that he had also been demonstrating signs of profound low mood and agitation. After discussion at a case review, the suggestion was made that Harry start cognitive behavioral therapy (CBT) and perhaps a course of antidepressants, but after discussion with Harry about his current medication it was revealed that he had been started on amiodarone, for an irregular heartbeat, 10 weeks before. Knowing that amiodarone is associated with depression, agitation and anxiety, the MHP referred Harry to the psychiatrist for a medication review and, rather than embark upon CBT or an antidepressant, the amiodarone was stopped and an alternative substituted. The depression and agitation resolved within a week or so and his anxiety returned to a moderate level without any further treatment being required.

Table 10.2 Psychological effects of some medicines prescribed for physical health

Medication	Prescribed for	Psychological effects
Propranolol	Hypertension	Depression, bad dreams
Simvastatin	Hypercholesterolaemia	Depression, tiredness
Amiodarone	Rhythm disturbances	Depression, psychosis
Aminophyline	Chronic Obstructive Pulmonary Disease	Anxiety, panic
Salbutamol	Asthma	Anxiety, panic
Corticosteroids	Asthma, rheumatoid arthritis	Depression, psychosis, delirium, mania
Methotrexate	Chemotherapy, psoriasis, rheumatoid arthritis	Depression
Omeprazole	Acid reflux	Depression
Isotretinoin	Acne	Depression, suicidal ideation
Penicillins	Antibiotics	Depression, agitation
Oral contraceptives	Contraception	Depression

CASE STUDY

SAFETY IN PREGNANCY

A final consideration is the potential adverse effects of prescribed medication on an unborn child, which is an area that tends to cause some anxiety for all involved in the care team. As with the sections above, the intention here is to assist in increasing the MHP's knowledge and awareness.

Seven per cent of mothers in their childbearing years suffer mental illness (NICE 2007). This, combined with the fact that 50–60% of pregnancies are generally 'unplanned' (NICE 2007), means that for many weeks the expectant mother may be potentially unaware of her pregnancy and consequently be unwittingly exposing her unborn child to psychotropic drugs.

The first step in facing this problem is an awareness of the risk. First trimester exposure is associated with abnormal organ formation and third trimester exposure is linked to withdrawal effects in the neonate – for example, the withdrawal seen with some antidepressants and antipsychotics. It should also be borne in mind that following birth babies may encounter any drugs that are secreted in breast milk.

Unfortunately, no drug can be deemed wholly safe. This means that a policy of avoiding drugs during pregnancy (especially in the first trimester) is the wisest course unless the risks posed to the mother by any relapse are severe and probable.

The following points are worth considering in planning an approach for women with mental health problems in their childbearing years. No guarantees about safety are available and there is a relative lack of research and certainty in this area.

When considering antidepressants, tricyclics are relatively safe in terms of any risk of malformations, but if used in the third trimester can lead to withdrawal symptoms in the neonate. There is less certainty about SSRIs and malformations. In relation to antipsychotics, phenothiazines are associated with a small risk of malformations, while haloperidol and olanzapine are considered safer. The mood stabiliser lithium is definitely associated with foetal cardiac abnormalities such as Fallot's Tetralogy, while valproate and carbamazepine are associated with neural tube defects. Finally, phenytoin is associated with facial cleft defects. To avoid problems with psychiatric drugs in pregnancy the following suggestions are made:

- In women of childbearing years prescribe drugs which are safer – just in case these patients become pregnant.
- Advise potentially fertile women with long-term mental health problems of the risks of medication and pregnancy and encourage planned pregnancies following discussion with the care team.
- Weigh up risks of using no medication during pregnancy or switching drugs to ones less associated with risk.
- Use scanning or other imaging for embryos exposed to potentially damaging drugs – this might lead to consideration of prenatal surgery for vascular abnormalities, neural tube defects or, sadly, termination in some cases.
- Folic acid supplements (used for neural tube defect prophylaxis).

CONCLUSION

After the daunting array of adverse effects and problems associated with the medication listed above the reader would be forgiven for wondering about the wisdom of prescribing any medication for mental health problems. There is without doubt a cost to the physical health of individuals who are prescribed these medications, but there is also a clear advantage – improved mental health. Despite the recent growth of psychotherapies, medication remains a major therapeutic tool, so it seems that MHPs are faced with a dilemma: whether to prioritise mental over physical health.

Perhaps the answer is to balance both, treating the psychological aspects while managing the physical. There are many ways that MHPs can minimise the adverse physical effects of psychotropic medication, but one of particular relevance to this topic is medication concordance. By taking a collaborative approach to minimising the potentially harmful effects of mental health prescribing, the service user is afforded the opportunity to take some control over their own health and wellbeing, which will not only enhance the chances of adherence for mental health treatment, but also that which is physical.

USEFUL RESOURCES

At the time of writing in the UK we recommend the following resources:

National Prescription Centre – www.npc.co.uk
British National Formulary – http://bnf.org/bnf/index.htm
Royal Pharmaceutical Society for Great Britain – www.rpharms.com/home/home.asp
Association of British Pharmaceutical Industries – www.abpi.org.uk/Pages/default.aspx
Association for Nurse Prescribing – http://anp.org.uk/
Drug Tariff Online – www.drugtariff.com/
Electronic Medicines Compendium – www.medicines.org.uk/emc/
Medicines and Healthcare Products Regulatory Agency – www.mhra.gov.uk/index.htm
www.nelm.nhs.uk/en/ - National Electronic Library for Medicines

11

PROMOTING PHYSICAL WELLBEING

CLARE STREET

Learning outcomes

By the end of this chapter you should be able to:

- Consider the impact of lifestyle factors on the physical wellbeing of the mentally ill
- Explore some of the difficulties and barriers to promoting healthy lifestyles
- Identify features of good practice and the implications for health and social care practitioners

---

INTRODUCTION

Many years ago, as a rather inexperienced health promotion officer, I was asked to do a session on 'smoking and health, and smoking cessation' for a group of mental health practitioners. To my surprise, they were completely disinterested, even hostile, and I was at a loss as to how to engage their attention. I had spent nearly two years working in acute medicine where I daily saw the serious and debilitating consequences of smoking, so my perceptions of the harms of smoking and the necessity of addressing this matter as a health concern were clearly at odds to this group of practitioners. According to Ratschen et al. (2011), this is still the case. This chapter will explore the evidence underpinning this area of practice and provide an overview of those health promotion strategies which have proved effective. In so doing, the chapter will present a clear case that those working in mental health should prioritise the promotion of physical health, which will hopefully contribute to the much-needed shift towards active engagement in the promotion of physical health, among people with mental health problems.

As discussed in Chapter 1, the case for promoting the physical health of people with mental health problems is compelling and this has become part of international western government priorities over the last decade or so. However, the challenge of implementing such improved practice remains, and this chapter will explore some examples of initiatives to provide insight into potential options for real-life practice. The focus will specifically be on modifiable lifestyle risk factors, given their high incidence and prevalence among people with mental health problems. Modifying these risk factors will have multiple health benefits.

THE IMPACT OF LIFESTYLE FACTORS ON PHYSICAL HEALTH

Lifestyle factors are regarded as contributing to the increased incidence and prevalence of coronary heart disease (CHD) and respiratory disorders. Smoking behaviour, obesity and lack of physical activity are particularly implicated in the aetiology of these diseases (Wildgust and Beary. 2010). Brown, Kim et al. (2010) consider smoking to be the biggest contributory factor in the excess of cardiac mortality among those with a severe mental illness (SMI). It is a known independent risk factor for a wide range of cardiorespiratory conditions and it considerably increases the risk of lung cancer (Joint British Societies 2005). There is a high prevalence of smoking among people with SMI, with rates of up to two to three times higher compared with the general population. Around 50% of these are heavy smokers (Banham and Gilbody 2010) and Faulkner et al. (2007) estimated that among people with schizophrenia this could be up to 90%.

Poor diet, including high sugar consumption, is also implicated in worse health outcomes for people with schizophrenia (Robson and Gray 2007), and an unhealthy diet and lack of exercise are linked to weight gain and a higher risk of diabetes (Brown, Leith et al. 2010). With regard to nutrition and health, the prime focus of attention is on cholesterol (for heart disease) and hypercholesterolaemia is a significant risk factor which can be treated with statins (Wildgust and Beary 2010).

Exercise and physical activity levels are frequently low among people with a SMI (Bobes et al. 2010; Weber 2010) and are implicated in the excess mortality experienced by this group (Oud et al. 2009). Physical activity is acknowledged to be protective against coronary heart disease and confers contemporaneous benefit, although these benefits cease when activity ceases (Joint British Societies 2005). According to Schmutte et al. (2009), the modifiable risk factors discussed account for nearly two-thirds of the 33% reduction in life expectancy of this vulnerable group.

Environmental conditions (poor housing, limited income, institutionalisation, social circumstances) also impact directly on health and lifestyle choices. Weiser et al. (2009) assert that a tripartite relationship between the mental illness (medication side-effects, lack of attention to physical symptoms or compliance with treatment), health-related behaviour (such as smoking, poor diet, lack of activity) and environmental conditions contribute to the increased risks and disease profile experienced by people with a SMI.

HEALTH PROMOTION WITH INDIVIDUALS WITH MENTAL HEALTH PROBLEMS

Apart from improving treatment and care options for those with physical health care needs, primary and secondary prevention remain important options too. It has already been noted that those with mental health problems have an increased susceptibility to conditions that are amenable to lifestyle change, such as smoking, physical activity and good nutrition (Wildgust and Beary 2010). There is evidence too that people with a mental health problem are interested in, and do respond positively to, health promotion information (Faulkner et al. 2007) and information about diet, dental health and how to remain healthy (Osborn et al. 2003). They are also receptive to encouragement to engage in smoking cessation, physical activity and general healthy lifestyle programmes (Schmutte et al. 2009). Therefore, risk reduction is possible (Cabassa et al. 2010).

Weiser et al. (2009) suggest that within most mental health facilities there is little experience of engagement with health promoting activity, and therefore structured support is essential. Strategies need to be developed that enable identification of health problems, appropriate interventions and the ability to evaluate outcomes (Weiser et al. 2009) and proactive training of practitioners is necessary. Robson and Gray (2007) call for greater clarity within and between health care providers regarding roles and responsibilities, and to monitor and address physical care needs and collaborative care planning across the multidisciplinary team. Advice on exercise and healthy eating, for instance, should be regarded as an integral part of routine care and active case management, and practitioner support is vital too (Mueser et al. 2006). Take a look at Action Learning Point 11.1.

Action Learning Point 11.1

- Having considered the modifiable risk factors for your clients, identify any health improvement/promotion strategies that you are aware of.
- How successful have these strategies been? Reflect on those factors which act to enhance or mitigate against the success of these strategies.

THE ROLE OF THE MENTAL HEALTH PRACTITIONER

This section will present an overview of the evidence on how engagement in health promoting activity might be established in practice. In particular, initiatives to promote smoking cessation, healthy eating and physical activity will be discussed. Given the nature of the risk factors, smoking is considered the main priority for change (Brown, Leith et al. 2010), but regardless of the specific focus of the lifestyle change/prevention programme, common principles of good practice emerge.

DEVELOPING SKILLS, KNOWLEDGE AND SELF-EFFICACY WITH SERVICE USERS

The development of skills and knowledge around health matters and the promotion of self-efficacy are fundamental to success. Active engagement is essential as there may be a mismatch between aspirations to engage in lifestyle change and perceived ability to do so among individuals with an SMI (Soundy et al. 2007). Schmutte et al. (2009: 4) note:

> Most participants wanted to learn more about healthy eating, exercise, and smoking cessation but felt doubtful about their ability to improve their health on their own.

Self-efficacy refers to an individual's confidence, belief and perceptions that they have the power to change their behaviour. It is linked with self-esteem but is based on a *realistic* assessment of achievement and expectations of personal success; in other words, 'How certain am I that I can do that?' (Thirlaway and Upton 2009). Self-efficacy influences all behaviour and is recognised as being the best predictor of behaviour change (Bandura 2002). Perceived self-efficacy will vary from 'task to task'. For example, an individual may have a high level of self-efficacy in terms of quitting smoking, but not for attempting to lose weight, and they will invest energy on the task and surmounting obstacles if they feel able to achieve their goals. Information alone does not contribute to success (Jones 2004). Rather, it is gradually attained by achieving competence, and building confidence, at each stage of a behavioural task or goal, such as successfully cooking a healthy meal (Baranowski et al. 2002).

According to Bandura (2000), people's sense of self-efficacy can be developed in four ways. These involve providing opportunities for using social persuasion (being told they can do it), vicarious experiences (seeing or being with others attempting to change), mastery experiences (i.e. improving an individual's skills and confidence), and providing experiences of success. Working to reduce people's stress reactions is also vital. The following case study provides an example of this process in action.

Tina

Tina was diagnosed with schizophrenia at the age of 22 and in the four years since she has gained a lot of weight. She has made several attempts to diet, but all have failed, and she feels she has no control over her spiralling weight. Tina's CPN suggests that she tries to increase her activity as a means of tackling her weight, but she is initially doubtful, saying that she lacks motivation. Her CPN gently challenges this by pointing out that she often walks to appointments and to meet friends, and he

(Continued)

CASE STUDY

(Continued)

suggests that she start by walking more as this is something she's proved she can do (social persuasion). He asks Tina if there is anybody she could go for walks with and she says her mother, who is also trying to lose weight (vicarious experience). Tina and her mother subsequently go on three walks to the local park, following which she reports feeling energised and positive (experience of success). Importantly, Tina's confidence in her ability to tackle her weight has increased and she is now thinking about walking further (mastery experience).

IMPLEMENTING HEALTHY LIFESTYLE SCHEMES

Examples of lifestyle change programmes involving individuals with mental health problems confirm the necessity of building self-efficacy by developing skills and providing opportunities for personal growth and autonomy. Active support is central to this achievement. For example, Shiner et al. (2008) observed that individualised interventions and positive and supportive interpersonal relationships, with a health mentor, facilitated participation in an activity and healthy eating programme (In SHAPE). Part of the programme involved arranging paid access to local fitness facilities but they noted that this alone was insufficient and it was the presence of the health mentor that enabled participants to feel confident enough to enter this setting. Simply being welcomed into the gym, being able to discuss progress and problems, enabled engagement. Appropriate goal-setting, practical advice, modifying food portion size, using incentives and organising group 'celebrations' all added to the positive impact of the programme and established mechanisms for the development of self-efficacy (Shiner et al. 2008).

Similarly, Bradshaw et al. (2010) discuss the development and evaluation of a health education programme aimed at changing 'risky' lifestyle behaviour among people diagnosed with schizophrenia. The programme structure and approach was based on the principles embodied in the trans-theoretical model of change (stages of change) (Prochaska and DiClemente 1986). The trans-theoretical concept of change is based on an understanding that change does not progress in a linear, ordered fashion, and that individuals pass through various 'stages' before they attain their change goal. One of the central principles of the model is that interventions need to be tailored to needs at specific points, and that the dynamic for change remains within the control of the individual. This emphasis helps avoid the problem of 'reactance', whereby people respond negatively and resist any change that they feel is externally imposed (Bradshaw et al. 2010).

The programme involved 10 one-hour sessions, and was person- and goal-centred, with an emphasis on problem-solving, peer support and practical advice. Taking account of possible attention and concentration problems, the sessions were structured around brief (20-minute) inputs and interactions. While attendance was variable, the programme was sufficiently flexible and person-centred for this not to undermine learning, and participant feedback indicated that they had enjoyed the social aspects of the group, found the peer support invaluable and commented that it had built their self-esteem. Participants also reported initiating several behaviour change or coping strategies as a result of participation in the programme, such as taking one cigarette, rather than the whole packet when they went shopping (Bradshaw et al. 2010).

A healthy living programme discussed by O'Sullivan et al. (2006) also incorporated a practical focus, such as visits to supermarkets, looking at food labels and nutritional content, selecting healthy food and providing assistance in preparing a meal. Whatever the nature of the lifestyle intervention, advice and action needs to be tailored to the individual and include realistic goal-setting and provide practical advice. In general, structured programmes are more likely to be effective, particularly those with peer support and a user focus.

SMOKING CESSATION

With regard to smoking, evidence suggests that this is an extremely important matter to tackle and people with a mental health problem do share a concern regarding this habit and are motivated to change (Johnson et al. 2010). Bobes et al. (2010) conclude that smoking cessation could reduce the excess death rate from CHD by 90%. The evidence suggests that it is possible to address smoking, although with modified parameters. For example, as Banham and Gilbody (2010) note, a primary goal of smoking *cessation* might not be realistic and it is suggested that *cutting down* on smoking (with or without nicotine replacement therapy) is a more achievable ambition. This fits with the principle of realistic goal setting, and the work of DiClemente et al. (2011) suggests that overall attainment of smoking cessation can be low (6.4% quit rate), but people with mental health problems are able to make general progress towards this goal.

In terms of specific interventions, Banham and Gilbody (2010) reviewed the evidence on smoking cessation therapy and concluded that the types of approach adopted for the general population are equally valid for those with mental health problems, particularly for those with a stable psychiatric condition, although additional, bespoke support increases the likelihood of success.

A combination of behavioural support and pharmacotherapy (nicotine replacement therapy (NRT), bupropion or varenicline) are generally most effective (Royal College General Practitioners and Royal College of Psychiatrists 2008; Banham and Gilbody 2010). According to Morrison and Naegle (2010), assessing motivation to quit and nicotine addiction (using the Fagerström Test for Nicotine Dependence (FTND), see Box 11.1) at the start of cessation efforts can be useful in order to tailor the intervention and support required, for example, indicating the potential need for pharmacotherapy.

Box 11.1 Using the Fagerström Test for Nicotine Dependence (FTND)

FTND is a brief, self-report questionnaire which identifies both physiological and behavioural dependence. Its current form (the FTND) is a revision of the original Fagerström Tolerance Questionnaire, developed by Fagerström in 1978 (Heatherton et al. 1991). Six questions are included, requesting information not only on the amount smoked,

(Continued)

Box 11.1   (Continued)

but also on patterns of smoking, such as how soon after waking the first cigarette is consumed and which cigarettes (e.g. the morning cigarette) would be most difficult to give up. These questions provide a score from 0–10. Scoring 7 out of 10 identifies the smoker as being highly dependent on nicotine, whereas as less than 4 is deemed to represent low nicotine dependence. High levels of dependency are judged to be associated with a greater likelihood of withdrawal symptoms on quitting. The FTND is easy to obtain and complete (literacy and access to the internet not withstanding) and an example can be found at www.outcometracker.org/library/FTND.pdf [accesed September 2012]

Motivational interviewing and work to promote a sense of self-efficacy are generally helpful too. Motivational interviewing seeks to establish a supportive relationship by directly acknowledging ambivalence around behaviour change and places the individual at the centre of decision-making, rather than the health professional in terms of goal setting (Davis et al. 2011).

Several studies have examined the use of group therapy, focusing on smoking cessation for individuals with SMI (Ashton et al. 2010; Griffiths et al. 2010). The Griffiths et al. (2010) study involved a 12-week, two-hour session, while Ashton et al. (2010) offered a 10-week group programme. Content of the programmes was structured, although flexible and client-centred, and differed in detail but included an emphasis on active goal setting, developing strategies to avoid triggers and pressures to smoke, and focusing on coping skills and relaxation exercises. Cognitive behavioural strategies to ameliorate negative thinking and time spent focusing on the positive aspects of reducing or quitting smoking, including financial benefits, also helped, along with efforts to promote self-confidence such as 'affirmation cards' (Griffiths et al. 2010). The success of smoking cessation interventions can be assessed either by the client's self-report or by checking expired carbon monoxide levels (Ashton et al. 2010). Although potentially paternalistic, this approach does offer a more objective measure of change.

Banham and Gilbody (2010), however, do signal a cautionary note regarding smoking cessation among people with SMI on two counts. First, while pharmacotherapy, particularly bupropion or varenicline, can enhance success, there are some reports of side-effects, with varenicline being linked to worsening mental health and bupropion lowering the seizure threshold. Consequently, bupropion should not be used in combination with some antipsychotics and antidepressants that have this potential too (McNally and The London Development Centre 2009), and the National Prescribing Service (2011) recommends NRT as the preferred option to support smoking cessation for people with SMI. The general advice is that NRT, bupropion or varenicline should not be used in any combination (NICE 2008), and the important factor in deciding between the pharmacotherapies is individual preference (NICE 2008).

Second, given the metabolic interaction between nicotine and antipsychotic medication, patients may require a reduction in antipsychotic medication as tobacco can reduce the serum concentration of antipsychotic medication (clozapine and olanzapine) by up to 40% (Johnson et al. 2010). Nicotine withdrawal itself can also mimic or exacerbate symptoms of mental illness, although Banham and Gilbody (2010) conclude that if someone was psychiatrically stable at the initiation of smoking cessation attempts, this did not adversely affect their mental health. Nevertheless, they recommend close monitoring and support for individuals.

A study being undertaken by Banham and Gilbody (2010), evaluating a bespoke service for smoking cessation support for those with SMI, is due to report in 2014 and this should add to our understanding of the effectiveness of such interventions. Overall, the literature on smoking cessation interventions for those with SMI indicates positive outcomes and what remains fundamental is 'sustained efforts in psychiatric settings to provide smoking intervention ... to enable SMI smokers to ... achieve cessation success' (DiClemente et al. 2011: 264).

PROMOTING PHYSICAL ACTIVITY

As Weber (2010) notes, exercise and physical activity are essential to address weight issues (alongside healthy nutrition), and for preventing metabolic consequences associated with diabetes. The positive effect of exercise on mood is well recognised and Iwasaki et al. (2010) report that exercise and leisure activities have a positive impact on those living with mental health problems. Additionally, there is evidence that physical activity helps to reduce the symptoms of psychosis, depression and anxiety among people with schizophrenia and improves subjective assessment of health (O'Sullivan et al. 2006).

Barriers to exercise, reported by people with mental health problems, include lack of motivation, lack of access to appropriate facilities and lack of transportation and the experience of sedation. However, simple exercise, such as a structured walking programme, has been both achievable and successful (reducing body fat and improving mental state) (Weber 2010).

Exercise regimes of some form or other are frequently incorporated into general healthy lifestyle programmes or linked explicitly with weight loss interventions. For example, Casagrande et al. (2010) discuss the ACHIEVE programme, which is currently at the trial stage (a randomised control trial) and incorporates intensive, structured, weight loss management sessions and group physical activity classes, within a mental health setting. At the pilot study phase, results have been positive in terms of weight loss and generally evidence suggests that any interventions aimed at changing lifestyle behaviour require active support in the context of a structured programme.

While there appears to be many positive opportunities for promoting activity among those with mental health problems, Voderholzer et al. (2011) and Hamera et al. (2010) note some limitations which need to be taken into account when designing activity programmes. Voderholzer et al. (2011) identified that seriously depressed patients had markedly low levels of physical fitness regardless of age or weight, and recommended careful measurement of baseline fitness to appropriately tailor the exercise regime to actual capacity. Fear of falling and personal injury among people with mental health problems is another concern, and in their study Hamera et al. (2010) noted balance difficulties in 40% of participants and muscular skeletal disorders in 30% of participants. Balance issues could justifiably influence ability and willingness to engage in exercise regimes so Hamera et al. (2010) recommend adjusting exercise programmes accordingly. This would include focusing on walking as a form exercise, particularly supervised walking at the initial stages, ensuring use of proper footwear and that the activity is confined to flat surfaces or pathways. Chair-based exercises may be an appropriate option too. An initial physical assessment and appropriate training in physical activity is important to reduce these risks (Casagrande et al. 2010). Now consider Action Learning Point 11.2.

Action Learning Point 11.2

According to Weber (2010), mental health practitioners should incorporate activity into their daily therapeutic work.

- How might you do this?
- What support and resources would you need?
- What other areas of work would you like to develop?

WEIGHT MANAGEMENT PROGRAMMES

Holt (2010: S195) challenges the 'therapeutic nihilism' associated with the treatment of obesity for those with SMI, and McCloughen and Foster (2011) draw attention to the significant impact weight gain (frequently induced by psychotropic medication) has on physical and psychological wellbeing, including increasing the likelihood of non-adherence to medication. Engaging with issues of weight gain is important at the outset of treatment with second-generation antipsychotics as this can be significant, up to a mean of 15.4 kg over two years (McCloughen and Foster 2011).

Motivation to control weight and knowledge of healthy eating is high among those with SMIs (Barre et al. 2011; McCloughen and Foster 2011). Although the specific evidence of effectiveness is often weak (lacking robust randomised control trial data), structured programmes do work and these do not have to be complex interventions (McCloughen and Foster 2011; Roberts and Bailey 2011). In a review of community-based interventions, Galletly and Murray (2009) noted that an intervention where participants were presented with food labelled 'green' (eat as much as you like), 'yellow' (eat with caution) and 'red' (stop before you eat) was among the most effective and add that this type of intervention might be the most appropriate given practical and resource limitations for both participants and practitioners.

Interventions involving active support from practitioners, using goal-setting strategies and personalised regimes tailored to the needs of the individual, have elicited positive results too (Barre et al. 2011; Hassapidou et al. 2011). Where possible, the involvement of family members and opportunities to prepare and consume healthy meals are also important (Barre et al. 2011).

Modifying drug regimes can also contribute to reducing or controlling weight gain. For example, co-administering olanzapine with reboxetine seems to diminish olanzapine-induced weight gain, as did the prescription of metformin (McCloughen and Foster 2011).

SHAPING THE ENVIRONMENT: PROMOTING PHYSICAL ACTIVITY AND HEALTHY EATING

Practical and environmental constraints may inhibit action and activity. For example, policies at places of residence may limit outdoor access, or the local environment (e.g. proximity to busy roads) may reduce opportunities for engaging in physical activity. Food choices and food availability too may encourage the consumption of foods high in carbohydrates and sugar, and limit access to fresh fruit and vegetables (Schmutte et al. 2009; Barre et al. 2011). Consequently, action to change local policy aimed at reshaping the micro-environment is vital to augment change (Barre et al. 2011). Knol et al. (2010), for instance, worked with small residential units to alter mealtime and vending machine choices, and to establish a group walking programme, and were able to make appropriate structural and operational changes. Think about Action Learning Point 11.3.

Action Learning Point 11.3

- What structural change may be necessary within your work environment?
- What action can you take to bring these environmental changes about?

CHALLENGES FOR THE MENTAL HEALTH PRACTITIONER

With regard to health promotion activities, socio-economic factors such as unemployment, stigma and poor social support may impact directly upon physical health and health-related behaviours too. Robson and Gray (2007) point out healthy lifestyle options might not be choices for many with a mental health problem, given the social, economic and environmental constraints they are likely to experience and depression, cost, lack of knowledge and confidence, and social isolation are likely to inhibit engagement in lifestyle change programmes.

Such activities are also unlikely to be popular among people with a mental health problem if they are restrictive or paternalistic (Weiser et al. 2009), and Schmutte et al. (2009) note that limited knowledge and feelings of powerlessness are likely to reduce engagement with change initiatives. Moreover, activities such as smoking are commonly regarded as having positive health outcomes too, such as reducing medication side-effects, improving coping mechanisms and improving psychological functioning (Weiser et al. 2009). Robson and Gray (2007) comment on practices within mental health care settings that reinforce behaviour such as smoking (via a reward system), and negative perceptions among health care practitioners of the capacity of an individual with a mental health problem to change their behaviour. These specific (and other general) normative beliefs and values associated with health-related behaviour have a strong influence on health-related behaviour choices and actions, and need to change (Ratschen et al. 2011). Changing normative practice is a challenge and requires structural and cultural shifts to ensure due priority is given to this work. Please see Action Learning Point 11.4.

Action Learning Point 11.4

- What barriers to change exist within your workplace?
- How might these be addressed?
- What support and resources do you need in order to change current practice?

An additional challenge is that attrition from these programmes can be high and actual attainment is often modest. For instance, Van Citters et al. (2010) found statistically significant results for changes in activity level (exercise, vigorous activity and walking) and reduced waist circumference, but not for weight loss, and the smoking cessation rates observed by DiClemente et al. (2011) were a mere 6.4%. Consequently, it could be claimed that these initiatives will not produce health improvements, raising doubts about the effectiveness/cost-effectiveness of such interventions.

However, there are many responses to this claim. First, practitioners should be striving to make initiatives effective by learning from their experiences, overcoming barriers and building on their successes. It can also be argued that health improvement is not just about the avoidance of disease and that there are many benefits from striving to modify lifestyle factors. Promoting autonomy, the fulfilment of potential and development of resilience are central to health (Seedhouse 2001) and Mueser et al. (2006) highlight social inclusion, meaningful activity, personal growth and responsibility, and hope as essential components of health too. Thus, judgements about the success of these lifestyle programmes should take account of their social and psychological benefits too (Knol et al. 2010).

Mueser et al. (2006) stress the value of emphasising subjective aspects of health improvement rather than just concentrating on specific 'disease prevention' targets and these *are* attainable outcomes. Shiner et al. (2008), for example, identified that participants reported increased levels of self-confidence, and normalisation of social activities as a consequence of involvement in a structured lifestyle programme. Offering opportunities for engagement and change is important in its own right and indeed may ultimately lead to tangible change and recovery through improved self-efficacy, engagement and perseverance (DiClemente et al. 2011).

Conversely, not providing these programmes would minimise opportunities for self (health) improvement and help maintain the status quo wherein the physical health needs of people with mental health problems are neglected. This, itself, would contribute to the continuance of the health gap experienced by those with mental health problems (Ratschen et al. 2011). Johnson et al. (2010) and Ratschen et al. (2011) argue strongly that normative practices which neglect physical health needs must be challenged and this will only change by active management and engagement with lifestyle change programmes and physical care programmes. Therefore, until this sort of therapeutic intervention becomes the norm, accepting that only a few may actively engage, and that prescribed outcomes are not always achieved (i.e. quitting smoking), may be a necessity. The evidence certainly points to general benefits gained by those who do take part and are supported in their ventures for change.

Additionally, health care is increasingly supposed to be person-centred (Department of Health 2011c) and if this is the case, many of the interventions discussed in this chapter certainly fulfil this requirement. So while questions regarding 'effectiveness' will remain, these sorts of interventions should become part of the established package of therapeutic care if the goal is to promote health for all (Ratschen et al. 2011). Take some time to think about Action Learning Point 11.5.

Action Learning Point 11.5

- What indicators might you use to judge success of these types of intervention within your practice?

CONCLUSION

In many ways the conclusions to be drawn from this perusal of issues and initiatives to promote the physical health of people with mental health problems are not surprising. They boil down to a commitment to address these needs, to provide a structure and environment within which these activities (including not smoking) become the norm, and require person-centred, active engagement and support. While this might seem prosaic, this is in many ways very positive as it is clearly within the capacity and skills of mental health and social professionals to actively engage with these health needs, thereby reducing some of the inequalities experienced by people with a mental health problem.

USEFUL RESOURCES

At the time of writing in the UK we recommend the following resources:

World Health Organization health promotion topic –
www.who.int/topics/health_promotion/en/
Public Health Agency UK – www.publichealth.hscni.net/
Institute of Health Promotion UK – www.ihpe.org.uk
International Union on Health Promotion and Education – www.iuhpe.org/
In addition, the Royal College of General Practitioners and Royal College of Psychiatrists (2008) have produced a useful leaflet on smoking cessation and mental health. This can be downloaded from www.mentalhealth.org.uk/publications/smoking-mental-health-primary-care/
For an interactive guide on pharmacology for smoking cessation go to:
www.nes.scot.nhs.uk/smoking1/index.html
This is designed for a pharmacy smoking cessation service but the information is nevertheless useful.

12

INFECTION PREVENTION AND CONTROL IN MENTAL HEALTH PRACTICE

JULIE HUGHES

Learning outcomes

By the end of this chapter you should be able to:

- Demonstrate an awareness of the basic principles of infection prevention and control
- List the risk factors for health care associated infection in patients with severe mental illness
- Discuss some of the challenges of infection prevention and control in mental health care settings

---

INTRODUCTION

Preventing and controlling infection is a vital component of health care regardless of the setting in which it takes place. The aims of all infection control strategies are to protect patients, staff and visitors from acquiring infection and to ensure that patients are cared for in a safe and clean environment.

Health care associated infections (HCAI) are high on the patient safety agenda due to increased morbidity and mortality and are a drain on health care resources worldwide (Department of Health 2006d, 2008; World Health Organisation 2009).

Although advancements in care and technology have improved patients' outcomes and prognosis, it has led to a patient population increasingly vulnerable to HCAI, e.g. Methicillin-resistant Staphylococcus Aureus (MRSA) and Clostridium difficile (see Box 12.1 for a definition of HCAI). In the UK, the Third National Prevalence Study of Hospital Acquired Infections identified that approximately 8–9% of patients acquire HCAI (Hospital Infection Society 2006). Newer infections such as H1N1 (swine flu), capable of causing pandemics, re-emerging infections (e.g. Mycobacterium Tuberculosis) and threats of biological terrorism all pose challenges for already stretched resources (Field et al. 2004; Fraise and Bradley 2009). Compliance with infection prevention and control (IPC) principles and procedures is a major factor in meeting such challenges and a key quality performance indicator. However, this can sometimes be suboptimal (Ott and French 2009).

Box 12.1   Defining HCAI

HCAI are infections acquired as a consequence of contact with any health care setting. They were previously referred to as Hospital Acquired Infections (HAI) (identified post-48 hours of admission) or Community Acquired Infections (CAI) (present on admission) (Silvestri et al. 2002; Fraise and Bradley 2009).

In response, there have been increasing national and international governmental directives aimed at reducing the burden of HCAI and ensuring that health care providers comply with IPC. In the UK this has included *The Health and Social Care Act: Code of Practice for the Prevention and Control of Health Care Associated Infections* (Department of Health 2009c). Service providers have to register with the Care Quality Commission (CQC), the regulatory monitoring body which has enforcement powers against poor or non-compliant organisations (Care Quality Commission 2008). The focus to date has been on acute health care organisations although mental health care facilities are now falling under increasing scrutiny. This is not surprising as although there is little current literature regarding HCAI among people with mental health problems, such individuals often have predisposing risk factors, including an increased prevalence of physical health problems than the general population (University of Manchester 2006; Waldrock 2009). They also pose challenges in complying with IPC, particularly in relation to isolation and self-hygiene often due to motivation, confusion, dementia and memory problems (Leggett and Williams 2000; Mackenzie et al. 2008; Hughes 2011). Furthermore, implementing IPC procedures can be difficult as necessary equipment such as soap, paper towels, alcohol hand rubs, clinical waste and sharps bins have to be carefully located to prevent risk of harm to self (e.g. ingestion or self-inflicted injury) or to others (e.g. using equipment as a weapons) (Leggett and Williams 2000; Hughes 2011).

WHAT ARE THE RISKS OF HCAI IN MENTAL HEALTH PRACTICE?

For infection to occur there have to be several factors involved, often referred to as the 'chain of infection'. Prevention of transmission of infection is dependent on breaking this chain (Bowell 1992) (see Figure 12.1).

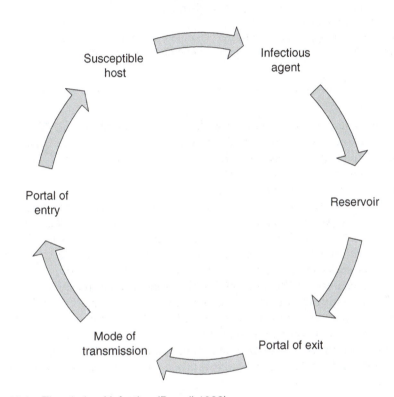

Figure 12.1 The chain of infection (Bowell 1992)

Factors predisposing patients to increased risk of infections can be found in Table 12.1. Wilson (2006) contends that individuals with mental health problems are clearly among those at increased risk. Not only are they often exposed to many of the factors identified (e.g. in-patient and residential care, poor hygiene, malnutrition or obesity and smoking), but they are particularly vulnerable to debility and disease due to lifestyle-related chronic diseases, as identified throughout the book. Increasingly, complex care is thus being delivered in community and mental health facilities, leading to less distinction between settings and more vulnerable patient populations susceptible to HCAI (Lawrence and May 2003; Blair 2009; Hughes 2011;).

Other risk factors associated with individuals with SMI include blood-borne viruses, sexually transmitted diseases and clients who self-harm, causing open

Table 12.1 Risk factors for infection

- History of hospital in-patient stay or other health care facilities, e.g. nursing and residential homes.
- Extremes of age (premature babies, frail elderly people).
- Family history of infection.
- Malnutrition or obesity.
- Poor personal hygiene, incontinence and general debility.
- Immune suppression due to therapy or underlying disease.
- Recent antibiotic therapy.
- Break in the skin (e.g. trauma, surgery, ulceration, trauma to tissues).
- Invasive devices (e.g. vascular or urinary catheterisation, surgical drains).
- Smoking.
- Metabolic disorders.

wounds which may become colonised with pathogens (Hughes et al. 2010). Finally, some antipsychotic medication can also lower neutrophils and affect gastric mobility, which are predisposing risks for the acquisition of infection (see Chapter 10 for further information on psychiatric prescribing).

Hughes et al. (2010) identified urinary tract infections (UTIs), lower respiratory infections and skin infections as the most common infections seen in mental health care settings. The main pathogens causing UTIs were found to be *Escherichia coli* (E Coli), in respiratory infections *Haemophilus influenza*, and for skin and wounds *Candida albicans* (thrush) and MRSA. Viral gastrointestinal infections such as norovirus can also cause outbreaks in such settings (Cheng et al. 2007). Interestingly, despite the formal implementation of IPC in mental health being a recent phenomenon, the first recorded major outbreak of food poisoning in a hospital was in a mental health facility in 1986 where several patients acquired *Salmonella* resulting in the UK National Health Service losing Crown Immunity (Murdoch 1992). Crown Immunity is a legal doctrine by which the sovereign or state cannot commit a legal wrong and is immune from civil suit or criminal prosecution. Now take a minute to consider Action Learning Point 12.1.

Action Learning Point 12.1

- Identify a client in your care and consider their risk factors in relation to acquiring a HCAI.

THE ROLE OF THE MENTAL HEALTH PROFESSIONAL IN PREVENTING AND CONTROLLING INFECTION

Although compliance with infection control policies can present difficulties in mental health care settings, the basic principles remain the same (Leggett and Williams 2000;

Hughes et al. 2010; Hughes et al. 2011a). Standard IPC precautions were developed in the 1980s and were originally referred to as universal precautions. They aim to provide health care workers (HCW) with guidance and regulations designed to prevent and control the spread of infection (Infection Control Nurses' Association 2002). Perry (2007) and Wilson (2006) identify the particular danger of HCW being exposed to blood or body fluids. Precautions apply to all body fluids, excretions and secretions, not just for clients known to have a blood-borne virus. As individuals' infection status is often unknown, IPC precautions are risk-based and should be applied in all areas of health care. This helps protect clients, staff and visitors and also prevents discrimination and the breaching of client confidentiality.

Universally accepted evidence-based standards for IPC include hand hygiene, use of personal protective equipment (PPE), safe handling and disposal of sharps, waste and linen, patient isolation, care of equipment, and environmental cleanliness (Infection Control Nurses' Association 2002; Pratt et al. 2007; Siegel et al. 2007; and the World Health Organization 2009).

THE IMPORTANCE OF DECONTAMINATING YOUR HANDS

Hand washing is acknowledged as the single most effective intervention to prevent the transmission of HCAI (Pratt et al. 2007; World Health Organization 2009), significantly reducing transmission of infection between patients, HCW and visitors. Unfortunately, it is often poorly performed and several studies demonstrate that compliance can be sub-optimal (Pratt et al. 2007; World Health Organization 2009). Reasons for this include availability of hand decontamination facilities, selection of harsh hand care products, workload and staff attitudes. The increased availability of alcohol handrubs has improved compliance (Pratt et al. 2007), resulting in a substantial reduction of transient micro-organisms. However, they are ineffective at removing physical dirt, soiling or the spore-forming bacteria, enteric pathogens, e.g. *Clostridium difficile* and norovirus. Further, frequent use may lead to product build-up where hands become 'sticky', due to the emollients used, which renders the product less effective. Therefore, hands that are visibly soiled or grossly contaminated with dirt or organic material must be washed with liquid soap and water which will remove transient micro-organisms, leaving hands socially clean. This level of decontamination is sufficient for general social contact and most clinical care activities. The technique for hand decontamination can be seen in Table 12.2 and Figure 12.2.

It is also important for staff to attend regular hand decontamination training sessions and audits. Policies should ensure that no jewellery, watches or rings (other than a plain wedding band) are worn, that nails are kept short and that acrylic/false fingernails and nail polish are prohibited to ensure effective technique (see Figure 12.3 for areas that can be missed by poor technique). Clinical staff should wear short sleeves (or long sleeves rolled up to above the elbow with no watches on the arm) when performing patient care procedures, i.e. the principle of 'bare below the elbow' (Department of Health 2010).

Table 12.2   Steps to effective hand decontamination technique

Step		Rationale
1	Remove all hand and wrist jewellery	To ensure that all surfaces of hand and wrist are able to be washed. To comply with Dress Code and 'Bare below the elbows'. Jewellery such as stoned rings and wrist watches limits the effectiveness of hand hygiene and can harbour micro-organisms leading to transmission. Nails should be short with no nail varnish/french manicure as this can become chipped when washing hands. Acrylic nails must not be worn as these have been implicated in the transmission of gram negative organisms.
2	Turn on taps ensuring water is at right temperature and correct flow	Prevents water being too hot or cold and helps minimise splashing of water to surrounding area.
3	Wet both hands thoroughly under warm running water before applying liquid soap	Prevents irritation and dry skin, which are more likely to support bacteria.
4	Rub hands together vigorously for a minimum of 15 seconds paying particular attention to tips of fingers, thumbs and areas between fingers (see Figure 12.2 How to hand wash)	Helps remove micro-organisms and ensures all areas are covered.
5	Rinse hands thoroughly under running water	Ensures that as much micro-organisms as possible are removed and no residues, which could contain micro-organisms/ cause skin irritation, are left on hands.
6	Turn taps off using elbows, wave motion or foot pedal. If none of these are possible, use paper towels to turn taps off	Prevents hands that have been washed becoming recontaminated with micro-organisms.
7	Dry hands thoroughly with good quality paper towels	Ensures that they do not provide an opportunity for further growth of micro-organisms. Disposable towels are recommended as they are single use and reduce the risk of recontamination.
8	Dispose of paper towels in accordance with local policy	Policies may vary locally. Some recommend disposal in bins suitable for household waste, while others suggest clinical waste containers.

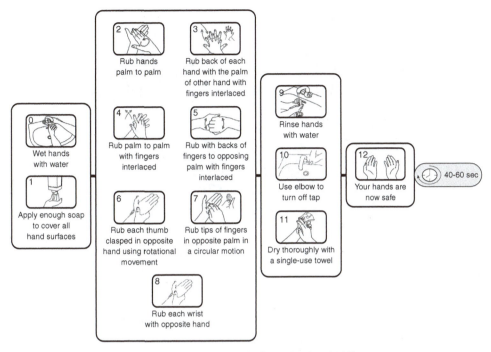

Figure 12.2   How to hand wash (World Health Organization 2009)

Source: Based on 'How to Handwash', www.who.int/gpsc/5may/How_To_HandWash_Poster.pdf
© World Health Organization 2009. All rights reserved.

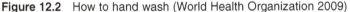

Hands must be decontaminated and dried thoroughly immediately before and after every episode of contact/care that involves direct contact with a patient's skin, their food, invasive devices, or dressings, and after any activity or contact that potentially results in hands becoming contaminated, such as contact with patient equipment and their immediate environment (further guidance from the National Patient Safety Agency, 'Your 5 moments for hand hygiene at the point of care' (2005, 2008) can be found in Figure 12.4).

Mental health practitioners should ensure that they apply hand cream in accordance with IPC policy to protect skin from the drying effects of regular hand decontamination and maintain skin integrity. Hands can become dry and sore, which has been shown to increase the potential for cross-infection of micro-organisms. Practitioners who do encounter skin problems must contact their Occupational Health Department.

Service users and carers play a crucial role in preventing the spread of micro-organisms (Hughes et al. 2011b). However, some individuals with mental health problems may be less likely to comply with self-hygiene due to motivation, confusion, dementia and memory problems (Mackenzie et al. 2008). Therefore mental health practitioners need to offer opportunities to encourage their clients to wash their hands.

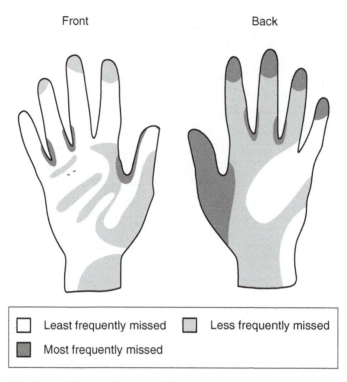

Figure 12.3   Areas most frequently missed by ineffective hand decontamination
Source: Taylor (1978) *Nursing Times*, www.nursingtimes.net

The National Patient Safety Agency (NPSA) 'Clean **your** hands' campaign (2005) encourages patients to become empowered around hand decontamination. Although this was initially focused at the physically ill, it has now been adopted in many mental health settings. There have, however, been cases reported of clients ingesting alcohol gel (NPSA 2008), reinforcing the need for each service to conduct and regularly review their risk assessment in relation to the placement of gel dispensers.

WHEN AND HOW TO USE PERSONAL PROTECTIVE EQUIPMENT

Personal protective equipment (PPE) must be worn to protect staff whenever they come into contact with clients' body secretions to reduce opportunities for transmission of micro-organisms (Infection Control Nurses' Association 2002). Employers have a duty to provide PPE for staff who, in turn, must wear PPE to comply with Health and Safety guidelines such as the Personal Protective Equipment Regulations (Health and Safety Executive 1992). PPE should be readily available and should always be based on a

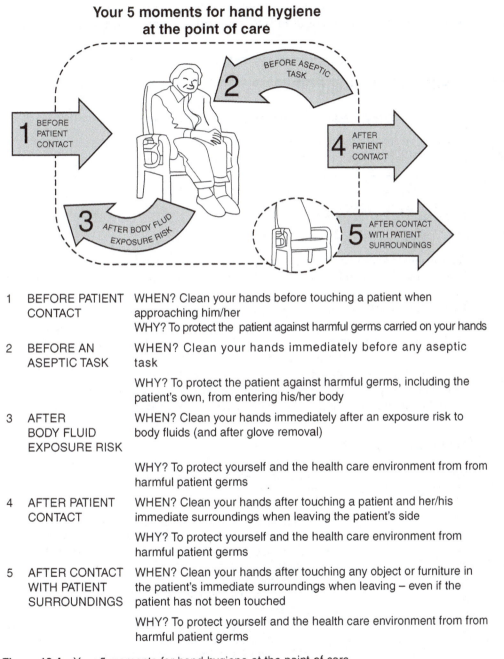

Your 5 moments for hand hygiene at the point of care

1 BEFORE PATIENT CONTACT
WHEN? Clean your hands before touching a patient when approaching him/her
WHY? To protect the patient against harmful germs carried on your hands

2 BEFORE AN ASEPTIC TASK
WHEN? Clean your hands immediately before any aseptic task

WHY? To protect the patient against harmful germs, including the patient's own, from entering his/her body

3 AFTER BODY FLUID EXPOSURE RISK
WHEN? Clean your hands immediately after an exposure risk to body fluids (and after glove removal)

WHY? To protect yourself and the health care environment from from harmful patient germs

4 AFTER PATIENT CONTACT
WHEN? Clean your hands after touching a patient and her/his immediate surroundings when leaving the patient's side

WHY? To protect yourself and the health care environment from harmful patient germs

5 AFTER CONTACT WITH PATIENT SURROUNDINGS
WHEN? Clean your hands after touching any object or furniture in the patient's immediate surroundings when leaving – even if the patient has not been touched

WHY? To protect yourself and the health care environment from from harmful patient germs

Figure 12.4   Your 5 moments for hand hygiene at the point of care

Source: Based on 'My 5 moments for Hand Hygiene', www.who.int/gpsc/5may/background/5moments/en/index.html © World Health Organization. All rights reserved.

patient and task risk assessment (see Table 12.3 for guidance on the use of PPE). Now consider your own use of PPE by completing Action Learning Point 12.2.

Action Learning Point 12.2

Reflect on current practice (yourself and your colleagues) and consider the following:

- Does it conform to the guidelines for hand decontamination and the use of PPE?
- If not, what factors act to prevent this and how might they be overcome?

ENVIRONMENTAL APPROACHES TO INFECTION PREVENTION AND CONTROL

A clean environment provides the background for good standards of hygiene and is an integral and important component of a strategy for preventing the spread of infection as well as maintaining the confidence of clients, staff and visitors (Department of Health 2004b). When considering the environmental cleanliness of in-patient settings it is vital that all staff are aware of their roles and responsibilities in keeping the environment clean. Increasingly, individuals with SMI receive care in the community setting where the focus is on creating a homely environment, which may be less conducive to optimum cleanliness. Furthermore, many people with mental health problems receive care in their own home and maintain control over their environment, which diminishes the influence of mental health practitioners regarding the levels of cleanliness.

Table 12.3 Use of PPE

PPE	When and why PPE should be worn
Gloves	Gloves must be worn:
	• To protect the hands from contamination with organic matter and micro-organisms or from sharp objects.
	• To reduce the risks of transmission of infection to both patients and staff.
	• To protect the hands when using cleaning products or when in contact with blood or body fluids, secretions or excretions.
	• When carrying out invasive procedures or when in contact with sterile sites, or non-intact skin or mucus membranes.
	• When cleaning during an incident of infection or an outbreak of infection.
	• When cleaning and using cleaning products.

PPE	When and why PPE should be worn
NB:	• Gloves are single-use item. • Put gloves on immediately before patient contact or treatment and remove as soon as the activity is completed. • Change gloves between caring for different patients and between different care treatments for some patients. • Gloves should not be worn for long periods. • Gloves must be removed carefully and hands decontaminated following removal. • Gloves must be disposed of as clinical waste. • All gloves should be latex free. • Sterile gloves should only be used for invasive procedures, when in contact with non-intact skin or aseptic technique.
Plastic Aprons	Aprons are provided for basic protection from blood or body fluids. Disposable plastic aprons must be worn when: • There is a risk that clothing may become exposed to blood, body fluids, secretions and excretions. • Clothing or uniform may be exposed to dirty conditions, e.g. cleaning, handling used laundry. Aprons must be changed and removed carefully: • Between care provided for each patient. • Between cleaning different areas, e.g. bedrooms, bays, toilets, kitchens and clinical areas. • During an outbreak of infection following cleaning of each individual room.
Gowns	Full body water repellent gowns must be worn when: There is a risk of potential gross contamination or extensive splashing of blood, body fluids, secretions and secretions on to the skin of health care workers. They are single-use only and dispose into clinical waste.
Masks	Must be worn: During an outbreak of infection where aerosol contamination is a risk, e.g. influenza and pandemic influenza or if a patient has open and active TB of the lung and is in the first 14 days of treatment. In this instance advice will be given on wearing FFP3 mask in the case of any aerosol-generating procedures. When using powder or toxic spray cleaning substances.
Eye Protection	Visors or goggles must be worn when: There is a risk of conjunctival exposure from blood or body fluids. Using powders, or when cleaning substances or toxic spray cleaning substances are used.

Clinical waste can present a particular challenge (Hoffman 2009). Clinical waste is defined as any waste arising from health care practice which may be toxic, hazardous or infectious and must be disposed of appropriately in accordance with the potential risk posed to patients, staff, visitors and the general public (Department of Health 2011d). Similarly, linen may become contaminated with micro-organisms from clients with infections or when soiled by blood, excreta or other body fluids (DH 1995; Hoffman 2009). Clinicians are thus advised to be aware of local policies with regard to the handling and disposing of clinical waste and linen, and PPE should always be used where there is a risk of contamination.

In mental health in-patient settings clients may be allowed to use washing machines to launder their own clothes. In this event, commercial machines, which are suitable for frequent use, should be used and they should be located in an area specifically designated for this purpose, ideally with a hand wash basin, and be on a pre-planned maintenance schedule. The machine should only be used for clients' own clothing, which should be laundered in individual batches to prevent possible transmission of micro-organisms. Contaminated laundry should not be washed by hand before placing in the machine as this poses the risk of aerosol dispersion and potential transmission. Linen should be tumble dried as it has been shown to further reduce microbial load.

The Case of Catriona below illustrates the importance of minimising the risk of cross-infection within an in-patient mental health care environment.

CASE STUDY

Catriona

Catriona is a 32 year-old woman who has a diagnosis of bipolar disorder. She has had several admissions to hospital over recent years, usually due to episodes of elation. During such episodes Catriona has a tendency towards promiscuity, which the staff are aware exposes her to the risk of acquiring sexually transmitted diseases and blood-borne viruses. This admission, however, is for severe depression and Catriona has not been attending to her personal care. Thus, she is presenting with malnutrition and poor hygiene.

Upon waking Catriona, the HCW finds that she has been incontinent of both urine and faeces and her bed and pyjamas are soiled. There is also evidence of blood on the sheets and it seems Catriona has been scratching her arms. Catriona is too unresponsive to attend to the situation and the HCW is faced with the following priorities: to protect Catriona's dignity, to assist to her hygiene needs, and to prevent contamination to staff and other clients. This is achieved by the mental health practitioner washing her hands and donning appropriate PPE (gloves and apron) before helping Catriona out of her soiled nightclothes. All soiled clothing is laundered without pre-soaking, and separately in line with the regulations. Catriona is covered up and escorted to the bathroom were she is assisted to wash and put clean clothes on (the clothes worn to get to the bathroom are laundered, as above). The HCW removes her gloves and apron before washing her hands. Upon returning to the bedside, Catriona is made comfortable in a chair and a new pair of gloves and apron are put on while the bed space is cleaned and the bed linen is removed and sent, in the appropriate coloured bag to identify it as soiled, to be laundered.

SAFE HANDLING AND DISPOSAL OF SHARPS

Many individuals with mental health problems will be prescribed intramuscular medications and will require regular venous blood sampling and/or blood glucose monitoring. As a result, those employed in mental health settings will require a working knowledge of the safe handling and disposal of sharps.

The central principles include wearing gloves when handling sharps as although this may not prevent an accidental exposure it can reduce the amount of blood inoculated. Sharps should be carried in a receptacle rather than by hand and should not be re-sheathed. It is the user of a sharp who is responsible for safe disposal so please remember: 'You use it – you bin it!' Sharps bins should be correctly assembled, not overfilled, and kept in a safe location at a suitable height – out of reach of clients and the public while in use.

Health workers are at risk of occupational exposure to blood-borne viruses and should be offered free immunisation for Hepatitis B prior to commencing employment, particularly those working on exposure-prone procedures and in high-risk areas, such as mental health (Infection Control Nurses' Association 2002). Occupational exposure can occur through the individual's failure to follow recommended procedures regarding the safe disposal of sharps and clinical waste. Accidental exposure is not, however, limited to needlestick injuries but also includes incidents when areas of broken skin or mucus membranes, such as the eyes and mouth, come into contact with blood or body fluids. Bites, scratches or spitting incidents may also occur in mental health settings and this represent a further risk of accidental exposure.

Incidents of accidental exposure are often under-reported (Murdoch and Cowell 1993) despite the prevalence of blood-borne viruses among people with mental health problems. In the event of an individual who is suspected or known to have a blood-borne virus, the risk to the recipient following a single sharps injury is estimated as follows:

- Hepatitis B – 33% (1:3)
- Hepatitis C – 1–3% (1:10–30)
- HIV – 0.3% (1:300)

Needles with hollow bores are also identified as a higher risk than other types of sharps.

Despite following safe working practices, accidents and malicious acts can occur, resulting in exposure to blood and body fluids and potential risk of infection. The case of Peter illustrates how a needlestick injury should be managed in clinical practice.

Peter

Peter is a CPN who is visiting Ajay at home to give him his depot injection. Peter has been visiting Ajay for a number of months and the procedure has become routine. Peter follows best practice when administering the injection by using a receptacle to carry the syringe (not disconnecting or resheathing the needle) and using a sharps bin for disposal. On this occasion, however, he is surprised to find that the bin is full, which he only realises when the needle falls out on to the floor. On retrieving this, Peter accidently pricks his finger with the needle. As he recognises this as a potential risk of cross-infection, he stops himself from acting on his first instinct, which is to put his finger in his mouth; instead asks Ajay if he can use a sink. Here he squeezes his finger, encouraging it to bleed and runs it under water. He ensures that the sink is left clean by wiping it down with kitchen roll and asks Ajay for a plaster. On his return to work Peter reports the incident to his manager and asks for more guidance. He is advised to contact the Occupational Health Department which will advise Peter about his options regarding screening.

Safe storage and disposal of sharps is essential in any health care facility. However, there is an acknowledged increased risk of sharps being used to self-harm in mental health facilities. In the event of a needlestick injury to a patient, the same procedure should be followed as for staff.

Another area of consideration is the risk of exposure to spillages of blood, urine and other bodily fluids. Local policies will provide detailed guidance in the use of PPE, isolation of the immediate area and cleaning procedure. In some instances, clients can deliberately contaminate their environment with body fluids (e.g. faecal smearing, which is sometimes referred to as 'dirty protests') or as a result of self-harm, which can lead to gross contamination of surrounding areas. In the event of this occurring, advice should be sought from the Infection Prevention and Control Team (IPCT) and specialist cleaning contractors may be brought in to decontaminate the area.

WHAT TO DO IF YOU SUSPECT A CLIENT OF HAVING AN HCAI

As discussed earlier, HCAIs are a significant risk to all in-patients and it is therefore appropriate to consider how best to care for susceptible individuals. In addition to standard IPC precautions, clients may be cared for in a side room if they are suspected of having a transmissible infection which could be of high risk to others (source isolation) or if they are particularly vulnerable to infection themselves, e.g. they are immunocompromised (protective isolation) (Kilpatrick et al. 2008).

The principles of client isolation include the following:

- Isolation precautions should be commenced on suspicion without awaiting microbiological confirmation.
- Clients should be placed in a single room with en-suite bathroom facilities.
- In the event of a single room not being available, a risk assessment with the IPCT should be undertaken.
- If two or more clients have the same infection (e.g. during an outbreak), it may be decided to cohort them in the same bay following advice from the IPCT.
- It is important to explain to the client why they are being isolated. This is important for any patient but is particularly important for those with mental health problems as it can affect their wellbeing.
- All clients should be risk assessed on a regular basis to identify when they no longer need to be cared for in a side room.
- The client's visitors should also be informed of any necessary precautions.
- Posters should be displayed outside the client's room to inform all those entering that this is an isolation area.
- Hands should be decontaminated before and after going into the side room.
- Use PPE and remove it before leaving the room, discarding it correctly.
- Following a patient risk assessment ensure that plastic bags used for infectious waste and linen are not stored inside the room as this has the potential to be used for self-harm.
- Disposable equipment should be used or if this is not possible then equipment could be designated solely for the patient.
- Domestic services must be made aware if you have clients with infections in your care.

THE PARTICULAR CHALLENGE OF COMPLYING WITH INFECTION PREVENTION AND CONTROL IN MENTAL HEALTH PRACTICE

Although the principles of infection prevention and control (IPC) are the same in all care settings, there are additional challenges to its application within mental health environments. The very nature of mental health care means that, as far as possible, the caring environment replicates the home environment in order to achieve a less institutional or 'clinical' care setting. Yet this poses a challenge to effective IPC as fixtures and furnishings may be more difficult to keep clean. Many potentially pathogenic micro-organisms (e.g. MRSA and norovirus) are transmitted via the environment and can result in heavy contamination of the care setting. Clients may also be encouraged to take responsibility for keeping their own area clean as part of the recovery process, but may feel less inclined or motivated to do so when unwell. They may also bring in personal belongings which can again lead to areas becoming cluttered and difficult to access or clean. In addition, ready access to cleaning solutions is more problematic due to the risk of potential ingestion, while body fluid spillages can also be a problem where clients may self-harm. A further challenge in the care of individuals who self-harm lies in the storage and disposal of PPE, which has the potential to be used to cause physical harm and should be kept beyond the reach of those individuals for whom it presents a risk.

Additional challenges face health care professionals tasked with caring for an individual with a mental health problem who is suspected of having an HCAI (Leggett and Williams 2000; Hughes et al. 2010; Hughes, 2011). The isolation procedures discussed earlier in this chapter identify that anyone suspected of having an HCAI should be cared for in the isolation of a side room. This may lead clients to feel anxious, low in mood and lonely as they are isolated from their peers. Some clients may be non-compliant (e.g. refusing to remain in the room) and becoming agitated, in which case the importance of being isolated needs careful explanation and it is likely that the individual will need additional emotional support during the period of isolation. Restricting a patient to a side room may be perceived as a form of restraint as it limits the individual's mobility and freedom, and HCWs should take advice in the event that a client is refusing this approach to treatment.

The situation is even more complex in the event that an individual with a propensity to self-harm is suspected of having an HCAI because PPE and clinical waste may need to be kept away from the client rather than in the room, which would usually be the case when caring for someone in isolation. Complete Action Learning Point 12.3 to identify the barriers to IPC in your working environment.

Action Learning Point 12.3

Consider the environment in which you deliver care and address the following questions:

- What factors may impede your ability to prevent and control infection for your clients?
- What strategies could you adopt to minimise these barriers?

CONCLUSION

Although the risk of HCAI is lower in people with mental health problems, they often have predisposing risk factors and it is important to ensure that all staff are fully conversant with the standard principles of IPC. This will help to protect clients, visitors and HCWs from largely preventable infections. However, complying with IPC precautions, guidance and legislation can be extremely challenging in this care environment. Mental health professionals have a key role to play in balancing the often competing need to care for their client's mental wellbeing, while also preventing and controlling infections among this vulnerable group. This is best achieved by adhering to IPC precautions, where possible, and adopting a risk-minimising approach where it is not. Effective liaison with IPC specialists is advised and should focus on assessing the risk of infection to all parties. Consideration should be afforded to the wider risks, such as self-harm or non-compliance. This should inform an individual care plan which incorporates the need for flexibility and allows for the holistic, person-centred approach at the very heart of contemporary mental health practice.

USEFUL RESOURCES

At the time of writing in the UK we recommend the following resources:

The Health Protection Agency UK – www.hpa.org.uk

European Centre for Disease Prevention and Control – http://ecdc.europa.eu/en/Pages/home.aspx

Reducing Healthcare-Associated Infections – http://hcai.dh.gov.uk

Infection Prevention Society – www.ips.uk.net

Centre for Disease Control and Prevention UK – www.cdc.gov

13

LEGAL AND ETHICAL MATTERS

MAUREEN DEACON

Learning outcomes

By the end of this chapter you should be able to:

- Work ethically and legally in the best interests of adult patients
- Understand the principal legal and ethical issues of health inequalities and discrimination, consent and capacity, and advanced care planning
- Discuss the matter of self-neglect and capacity

INTRODUCTION

In this chapter I discuss three main legal and ethical issues: health inequalities and discrimination, consent and capacity, and advance care planning. The chapter concludes with ideas about the attributes that a mental health practitioner requires if they are to work ethically and legally in relation to the physical care of the mentally ill. Where the law is examined in detail, I refer to that providing for England and Wales. However, the arising principles and debates have international resonance and readers are encouraged to learn more about the legal frameworks in their own national settings.

Consideration of ethical and lawful practice is primarily aimed at encouraging careful decision-making, which is the basis of accountable practice. While lawful practice is strictly rule governed, allowing only for limited, local interpretation, ethics deals with moral alternatives (Thompson et al. 2006). Whichever context takes precedence, difficult decisions will always have to be taken and it seems right and proper that mental health practitioners should struggle with moral dilemmas. 'Easy' decision-making implies a lack of thought and unjustified assumptions. Critical and morally-mature practitioners may sometimes have sleepless nights.

HEALTH INEQUALITIES AND DISCRIMINATION

That people with severe mental illness (SMI) have greater morbidity and mortality than the general population is accepted as a disturbing aspect of health inequalities; indeed, this has been reported for decades (Leucht et al. 2007). This matter has been examined in relation to specific disease processes in the preceding chapters and the reasons for this phenomenon have been discussed. These reasons can be broadly summarised as those relating to the person's mental ill health, for example, the administration of psychotropic medication may lead to weight gain, which, in turn, may impact adversely on cardiovascular health (McCloughen and Foster 2011), and those salient to the experience of health care. The latter have been referred to as a form of structural discrimination (Howard et al. 2010).

Within the field of bio-ethics it is argued that justice demands that policy-makers and practitioners should work to combat unjustified health inequalities. Francis (2007) notes that while practitioners' work is ethically contextualised by powerful organisational matters, such as resource constraints, they still have the responsibility to make ethical decisions at an individual level. This ethical decision-making is practised against the background of an interpretative and moral conceptual framework and it is this that needs to be articulated and challenged if these inequalities are to be eradicated. Next I will investigate some examples of this discriminatory background.

First, we can consider the mental health practitioner who does not believe that the physical health care of their patient is their concern or responsibility. This will have consequences for matters such as the facilitation of healthy nutrition, taking up and managing health screening opportunities, taking patients' health concerns seriously and enabling their further investigation, the provision of evidence-based health care interventions and communicating with other health care organisations. The absence of these health promotion strategies can be regarded as discriminatory against the mentally ill because patients in other health care settings can expect these interventions as normal practice. Leucht et al. (2007) are critical of psychiatrists who do not use their extensive physical health care skills and recommend urgent skill updating.

Second, patients may experience diagnostic overshadowing when they raise concerns about their health. Jones, Howard and Thornicroft (2008) discuss the complexity of this phenomenon and note how its presence in different 'minority groups' has been researched. They argue that a more accurate term is 'diagnostic and *treatment* overshadowing', given some research findings. For example, a study found that African-American women were less likely to be referred for cardiac catheterisation than white men, despite evidence of the same clinical need. The basis of overshadowing may be related to difficulties in communication, difficulties in complex diagnostic understanding, stereotyped ideas about the presentation of particular groups or prejudice and stigma. It may also relate to the patient's previous presentation. Consider the case of Jenny.

CASE STUDY

Jenny

Jenny has a diagnosis of borderline personality disorder and has suffered from several episodes of moderate/severe depression. When depressed she can become preoccupied with her physical health and frequently attends her family doctor with physical complaints, worrying that they are signs of cancer and subsequently requesting investigations. Over the years she has had many physical investigations all returned as normal. It is not uncommon for her to focus on particular symptoms and she frequently complains of abdominal pain and constipation. Recently she has added a new complaint of a frequent need to pass urine. Routine analysis has not revealed any abnormalities, nor is she pregnant and her doctor persuades her to keep it 'under review'. She may, of course, have a serious health problem, ovarian cancer for example, in which case she needs diagnosis and treatment as a matter of urgency, but we can understand why the doctor is using delaying tactics in the context of her previous presentations.

Jones, Howard and Thornicroft (2008) express the view that our understanding of diagnostic and treatment overshadowing with the mentally ill population is very limited and they argue for further research in the field.

Third, health care practitioners may make unjustified and incorrect assumptions about patients' needs and wishes (Dimond 2008). We may assume, for example, that because Fred's personal hygiene tends to be poor that he is not interested in having his teeth looked after, or that because Florence is chaotic, deluded and strangely dressed that she is not concerned about being obese and having very heavy menstrual periods. Such assumptions, which can lead to neglect and consequent health problems, can be regarded as matters of discrimination, that is, unjustified differential treatment (Francis 2007). Practitioners may be both subtly and overtly influenced by their personal and cultural values concerning the components of a good life and make judgements based on assumptions that a disabled and/or chronically ill life is necessarily an inferior one (Francis 2007). Before moving on, consider Action Learning Point 13.1.

Action Learning Point 13.1

- Discuss confidentially with a trusted colleague your personal views, judgements and feelings about the lives of people who have severe and enduring mental health problems. Consider the evidence you have for these views and how they may affect your motivations in caring for people. If you find it a useful learning strategy, you could go about this by writing reflectively.

The discussion thus far has focused on the attitudes of others to people with SMI and the likely consequences of these health inequalities. Now I turn to the person with SMI and their ability to give informed consent to care and treatment.

CONSENT AND MENTAL CAPACITY

Health care and treatment may not be given to patients who have mental capacity (sometimes referred to as competence) without their informed consent. To do otherwise is considered as 'trespass to the person' (Dimond 2008). This is an accepted ethical and lawful principle. Brock (2007) states that robust informed consent is made up of giving patients information in a form which they can understand, ensuring that consent, if given, is given voluntarily and that the person giving consent has the mental capacity to so do. Largely this process is routinely and successfully managed within health care organisations in both straightforward and highly complex cases. However, the mental capacity to give informed consent may be extremely problematic in some cases and ethical questions may arise when people make 'unhealthy' choices. Savulescu (2007) argues that competent people have the right to make autonomous, if controversial, choices. Just how controversial such choices are judged to be is a matter of context and social and cultural norms. As Dimond (2008: 10) states:

> It is a basic principle of the common law that a mentally competent adult is able to refuse even life saving treatment, for a good reason, a bad reason or no reason at all.

Mental health practitioners tend to be very familiar with lawful matters of consent and capacity as they relate to mental disorder. The law in this field is long established and has evolved historically. In contemporary times this international evolution has largely concerned further protection of patients' rights and moves to enforce treatment regimes on patients residing in the community. These changes have been strongly contested on ethical and practical grounds. In England and Wales, for example, it took 10 years to amend the Mental Health Act 1983 to become the Mental Health Act 2007 (Barber et al. 2009a).

The mental capacity to consent to physical care by the mentally ill is not covered by the Mental Health Act 2007 (Department of Health 2007; Dimond 2008) but is covered by the Mental Capacity Act 2005 (Department of Health 2005a) (again this relates to England and Wales). Note that treatment for mental disorder is not covered by the Mental Capacity Act 2005. The latter took more than 15 years of work to be passed and was prompted by action from the Law Society, which had highlighted the fragmented and out-of-date nature of the law at that time (Brown et al. 2009b). Dimond (2008) had argued that the untested and confusing relationships between the Mental Health Act 2007 and the Mental Capacity Act 2005 would lead to further amendments over time and this accurate prediction is discussed further below.

The Mental Capacity Act 2005 (MCA) is accompanied by a Code of Practice (Department of Health 2005c) and both these documents are easily accessible (see recommended resources below). The main purpose of the MCA is to provide a statutory framework for decision-making in the interests of adults who lack mental capacity. Its provisions are underpinned by two main concepts: capacity and best interests. The law assumes that all adults have mental capacity unless it is established that they do not. Moreover, it establishes that mental capacity should only be judged in relation to specific matters; this is often referred to as 'functionality'. Thus we may be capable of making some decisions but not others. Mental capacity is judged by a two-stage test. In the first stage it is established that the person:

> ...is unable to make a decision for himself [sic] in relation to the matter because of an impairment of, or a disturbance in the functioning of, the mind or brain. (The Mental Capacity Act 2005: Part 1 (see Department of Health 2005a))

The second stage is concerned with judging if this impairment or disturbance results in 'an inability to make or communicate decisions' (Dimond 2008: 34). When mental incapacity has been established, the decision-maker, in law, has to make decisions in relation to the person's best interests. However, advance decisions or specific instructions contained within Lasting Power of Attorney documentation take precedence, even if they may not be in the person's best interests. The context in which the person's best interests should be considered is set out in the MCA (section 4). It includes, for instance, the responsibility to consult and take account of the views of carers and loved ones. If they can demonstrate that the relevant matters have been attended to in decision-making, the decision-maker is protected by the Act. The MCA does not set down who has the legal right to be a decision-maker. Decisions about patients being cared for in health care and social care settings should be made by appropriate professional staff. When disputed decisions cannot be resolved by those involved with the patient, then an application can be made to the Court of Protection. It appears to be assumed that this will happen rarely.

The MCA also makes provision for the appointment of an Independent Mental Capacity Advocate (IMCA) in 'serious' cases where there is no appropriate person to consult with. Serious cases refer to decisions about serious medical treatment (e.g. major surgery) and moving a person into residential/nursing home accommodation.

Dimond (2008) has made the important observation that in mental health services it is often only when a patient disagrees with a proposed psychiatric intervention that their capacity is questioned. We can speculate whether this will follow too in relation to physical care.

The Mental Health Act 2007 amended the MCA to include Deprivation of Liberty Safeguards (DoLS). Their purpose is to legally deprive a person lacking capacity of their liberty within a care home or hospital in their best interests. Essentially it allows for the lawful protection of such people. It was envisaged that the DoLS would be used for people with dementia, severe learning disability and neurological conditions. The DoLS procedure includes that the intention to deprive someone of their liberty must be set out in an application to a supervisory body – the bodies that have regulatory authority for health and social care residential services. The application must be made by the 'Managing Authority', this being either the NHS authority where the person is to reside or, in the case of a private hospital or care home, the person registered to carry out this role. The supervisory body must then make an assessment of the person and recommend whether or not to grant authorisation. Enforced from 1 April 2009, the use of the DoLS is gradually increasing in England. The data available thus far shows a higher proportion of authorisation for women and for those residing in local authority care (Health and Social Care Information Centre 2011). The former presumably reflects women's longer lives and the latter the policies of care provision in England. A DoLS authorisation can last up to one year and appeals against authorisation can be made to the Court of Protection.

While in the main the MCA has replaced common law, there are two areas of such law left over: being able to act in emergency situations when the application of lawful procedures is impractical; and intervening to prevent a person from harming someone else.

The relationship between the MCA and the Mental Health Act is complex and potentially confusing and clearly this is of great importance when deciding about the best legal framework for effective care and treatment (Brown et al. 2009b). Now I will turn to considering the physical care of a person detained under the Mental Health Act 2007 and the interface with the MCA by looking at the case of Elizabeth.

Elizabeth

Elizabeth, aged 64 years, is suffering from severe depression. She is being detained and treated in hospital under the Mental Health Act 2007. Elizabeth is severely agitated and has depressive delusions. She believes that she is impoverished financially, has committed heinous acts and is guilt-ridden. She is constipated following a long period of appetite loss and consequent poor nutrition. She believes that her 'bowels are blocked up with toilet paper'. One morning she is observed to be very pale and clammy and appears to have acute abdominal pain. Her pulse is rapid and thready. She refuses to let the psychiatric staff examine her further, claiming that she is being punished by God.

Elizabeth's psychiatrist, Sue Jones, would like her to be assessed as a matter of urgency by a surgeon. The Mental Health Act only makes provision for the treatment of mental disorder and Dr Jones does not think that her physical distress is linked to her depressive illness. In this case Elizabeth needs to have her capacity assessed in relation to surgical examination and, potentially, consequent treatment. Dr Jones (in this case initially being the decision-maker) and Elizabeth's named nurse, Jacob Kobi, apply the two-stage test and establish that she: '...is unable to make a decision for himself [sic] in relation to the matter because of an impairment of, or a disturbance in the functioning of, the mind or brain' (The Mental Capacity Act 2005, Part 1) and that she is unable to make a decision because of this mental incapacity. They are firmly of the view that

(Continued)

CASE STUDY

(Continued)

an urgent surgical consult is in her best interests. While Dr Jones contacts the on-call surgical team, Jacob contacts Elizabeth's husband, informs him of the current situation and seeks and receives his approval of their actions. He clarifies that there is no person with Lasting Power of Attorney in place. On arrival at the ward, the surgeon finds Elizabeth in her bed area but she is refusing to be examined. Like his colleagues the surgeon can see that she looks acutely unwell and is of the view that she lacks capacity. He realises that she will have to be restrained in order that his physical examination can take place and he acts as the decision-maker to request that this takes place. The MCA makes provision for restraint and defines it as: '(i) the use or threat of force in any action which the person resists, or (ii) any restriction of a person's liberty of movement, whether or not they resist'. The surgeon may authorise restraint because he 'reasonably believes that it is necessary to do the act in order to prevent harm ... and that the act is a proportionate response...'

Elizabeth is examined while being restrained by Jacob, Dr Jones and two health care assistants. The surgeon prescribes injectable opiate analgesia and a benzodiazepine which relieves her pain and has a sedative effect and later Elizabeth undergoes abdominal surgery. The surgeon, Sue Jones and Jacob Kobi account for the decision-making process as it relates to the MCA in Elizabeth's health record. Some organisations may have developed specific documentation for this purpose.

The use of the DoLS is relatively recent and we can expect case law to develop in this area. Now consider Action Learning Point 13.2.

Action Learning Point 13.2

- Investigate the law relating to mental capacity/competence within the jurisdiction where you work.
- Imagine some alternative cases and work through how the law would be applied in real-life practice.

SELF-NEGLECT AND CAPACITY

Self-neglect poses particular challenges to the person's health and the ethics of autonomy. It has received far less attention than the more dramatic risks of violence and suicide by the mentally ill. Many people live in varying degrees of squalor and have poor personal hygiene. The exact point at which intervention should be considered is impossible to state without a full picture of the context in which self-neglect is occurring. For example, Jackson, aged 82, who has early Alzheimer's disease, has, according to his three younger sisters, always lived in 'dirty and disor-ganised chaos', whereas Ann, of similar age and stage of dementia, has always been meticulous in her appearance and housekeeping but latterly has stopped bathing, cleaning her home and washing her clothes. The MCA 2005 Part 1 (Department of Health 2005a) can provide a framework for decision-making in these fictitious cases of self-neglect. Its five principles are:

1 A person must be assumed to have capacity unless it is established that he lacks capacity.
2 A person is not to be treated as unable to make a decision unless all practicable steps to help him do so have been taken without success.
3 A person is not to be treated as unable to make a decision merely because he makes an unwise decision.
4 An act done, or decision made, under this Act for or on behalf of a person who lacks capacity must be done, or made, in his best interests.
5 Before the act is done, or the decision is made, regard must be had to whether the pur-pose for which it is needed can be as effectively achieved in a way that is less restrictive of the person's rights and freedom of action. (The Mental Capacity Act 2005: Part 1)

Using these principles, Ann's social worker and family decide that though Ann does lack capacity in this context (on the basis that she has a diagnosis of dementia and is behaving in sharp contrast to her pre-morbid state), she is willing to allow carers into her home to give her a bath every day and for her family to clean her house and do her laundry. Returning to Jackson, he has several badly infected leg ulcers, which are malodorous and seemingly painful, but he is refusing to allow them to be assessed or treated. His explanation is that he will not have 'strangers' in his house. Now consider Action Learning Point 13.3.

Action Learning Point 13.3

- What matters would you take into account when applying the five principles to Jackson's case?
- At what point might you consider the use of the DoLS?

Had Ann or Jackson been involved in advance care planning the decisions made could have been better informed.

ADVANCE CARE PLANNING

The idea that people should be encouraged to plan for a time when they no longer have the capacity to make important decisions for themselves has gained policy momentum in contemporary times. We can speculate that this is related to various issues: ageing societies; the growth of life-limiting but long-term conditions in the industrialised world; ethics that have challenged paternalistic health services; and an emphasis on person-centred care. No doubt people have always had private views about their future care, but today these matters are being written into legislation internationally. However, advance care planning (ACP) can result in the general ability to have one's wishes taken into account and/or be part of a formal, legal process. As Brock (2007) argues, the more controversial a decision is: particularly if it is likely to have negative health consequences, the more likely we are to expect high level decision-making capacity. I will examine how this can have ramifications with different types of advance care planning.

In the UK, the National Health Service and the University of Nottingham (2008) describe four activities that can be considered: (1) ACP; (2) a written statement of wishes and preferences; (3) advance decisions; and (4) the role of Lasting Power of Attorney. The latter two are provided for in the MCA.

Advance care planning is a process of contemplation and communication in which a person with capacity makes decisions about their future health and/or personal care in the event that they become incapable of giving informed consent. The process may involve discussions with significant others and health care providers. This activity is likely to arise in the context of developing a life-limiting condition, so clearly the person will benefit from a good understanding of that condition, its treatment, its prognosis and what may happen to them. It makes sense that these plans should be documented, made known to likely advocates and reviewed from time to time. These plans could be written as a statement of wishes and preferences and could include statements about the person's values that would guide their decision-making. Communications from ACP and written statements are not legally binding but should be taken account of when making surrogate decisions about the person's best interests. While these processes have mainly been considered in relation to end-of-life care (e.g. in dementia and terminal cancer), there is no reason why they cannot be used for people with severe and enduring mental illness who are likely to relapse in the future. This is discussed further below.

Legally, advance decisions are made to refuse specified medical care in the circumstances that the person has lost capacity to consent. They can only concern refusal of a specified medical treatment by a health care provider. So, for instance, a person can refuse IV antibiotics in the event that they are unconscious and have a chest infection but they cannot demand to die at home. The latter will be taken into account but will not be legally binding. Barber, Brown and Martin (2009b) note that a person cannot refuse in advance basic care, including nursing care. Under the MCA an advance decision is only effective if it is 'valid and applicable'. It will not be valid if the person has changed their mind and withdrawn it (assuming that they have the capacity to do this) or if the person acts erratically. For example, a person makes an advance decision to refuse chemotherapy for advanced cancer but three months later accepts it, having the capacity to make such decisions. If a person makes a Lasting Power of Attorney following an advance decision, then the latter is normally superseded by the former.

To be applicable the advance decision must clearly specify the treatment to be refused and the person must lack capacity when it is being used. Despite its legally binding nature, the formal rules about advance decisions are quite woolly. For instance, it can be given verbally or in an undated statement. The exception to this is in the case of the refusal of life-sustaining treatment, where the person has to give a written statement which is signed and witnessed, and stating that it should apply even if their life is at risk (Barber et al. 2009b). The MCA Code of Practice (9.19) (Department of Health 2005c) makes helpful suggestions regarding the presentation and communication of advance decisions. Now consider Action Learning Point 13.4.

Action Learning Point 13.4

- Consider the circumstances in which you would choose to engage in advance care planning.
- Discuss your views on not providing life-sustaining treatment in the context of a valid and applicable advance decision.
- Investigate policy and law relating to advance care planning within the jurisdiction where you work.

As previously noted, the public discussion about ACP has been largely in relation to end-of-life care and dementia. However, it is a matter that has also been considered in the case of people with severe mental illness whose capacity may fluctuate (Papageorgiou et al. 2002). Swanson et al. (2006) studied the use of a structured intervention to support people with SMI (who had capacity) to engage in ACP. Participants, for example, stated preferences for, and refusal of, particular drugs. It was found that the participants reported better working relationships with their care team and were more satisfied with their treatment. However, Papageorgiou et al. (2002) found that the use of ACP did not have an impact on hospital length of stay, although I argue that this is just one potential outcome. Ultimately, treatment decisions made using the Mental Health Act 2007 would take precedence over the patient's ACP, but this could only ensure that the mental health team's decisions were robust and transparent.

If a person with SMI has a co-morbid physical health problem, then clearly it would be to their advantage to include this in ACP too. In practice, there may well be a situation where a patient has made various advance care plans, some which are legally binding, some which are not. Let us consider the case of Joan.

Joan

Joan, aged 51, has recently been diagnosed with early-onset dementia. Five years ago she was successfully treated for early-stage breast cancer. With the support and

(Continued)

CASE STUDY

(Continued)

encouragement of her family and community mental health nurse she engages in advance care planning. First, she makes an advance decision that if she loses capacity and develops secondary breast cancer she refuses all cancer treatments with the exception of palliation. Joan clearly specifies that she is refusing all forms of chemotherapy and surgery. The nurse, with reference to the MCA Code of Conduct, ensures that Joan makes this advance decision correctly and that copies of her statement are lodged appropriately. Joan asks her husband and daughter to take on the role of Lasting Power of Attorney and together they complete the paperwork managed via the Office of the Public Guardian. Joan has always been a fastidious person in relation to her appearance and her home, and she has always had a pet cat. She makes a statement of her wishes concerning her care should she lose capacity.

Given a person's desire and willingness to engage in ACP, it is a highly ethical process as it promotes autonomy, choice and adherence to the person's best interests.

CONCLUSION

To work ethically and lawfully in caring for the physical health of a person with a SMI the mental health practitioner needs the following:

- A commitment to physical health care and the rights of the SMI to expect care which promotes their physical and mental health.
- Knowledge of the law and the local processes for its implementation.
- The motivation to learn about unfamiliar health problems to the advantage of individual patients.
- The confidence to communicate about sensitive matters with patients and their loved ones.
- The confidence to communicate with unfamiliar health care and social care professionals working within unfamiliar settings.
- The determination to advocate for patients' best interests in the face of discrimination, diagnostic and treatment overshadowing, health inequalities and in the case of incapacity.
- The ability to promote organisational change and develop practice.
- The development of self-awareness concerning personal values about the moral worth of different lives.
- This can be summarised as working with the patient in their best interests whether they have capacity or not. Where a patient lacks capacity, Brock (2007: 138) defines best interests thus: '...the decision that most reasonable persons will make in the circumstances'.

The Code of Practice for the MCA (Department of Health 2005c: Chapter 5) sets out a 'checklist' for best interest decision-making: encourage the person's participation;

identify all relevant circumstances; identify the person's views; avoid discrimination; assess whether or not the lack of capacity is permanent; consult others; do not be motivated to bring about the person's death; and use the least restrictive options possible.

To work ethically and within the law are routine social expectations of mental health practitioners. While undoubtedly challenging, accountable practitioners have the power and compassion to make a positive contribution to the difficult times of people needing care.

USEFUL RESOURCES

At the time of writing in the UK we recommend the following resources:

Department of Health (2005) *Mental Capacity Act 2005 Code of Practice* – www.dh.gov.uk

Department of Health (2009) *Mental Capacity Act 2005: Deprivation of Liberty Safeguards – Code of Practice Supplement to the Main Mental Capacity Act 2005 Code of Practice* – www.dh.gov.uk

Department of Health (2009) *Mental Capacity Act 2005: Deprivation of Liberty Safeguards: A Guide for Hospitals and Care Homes* – www.dh.gov.uk

Department of Health (2009) *Reference Guide to Consent for Examination or Treatment* (2nd edn) – www.dh.gov.uk

Department for Constitutional Affairs, Department of Health and Welsh Assembly Government (2005) *Mental Capacity Act Easy Read Summary*. London: HMSO (potentially useful for people with learning disability)

For very useful information for patients and carers suffering from Alzheimer's disease – www.alzheimers.org.uk

Social Care Institute for Excellence – www.scie.org.uk

GLOSSARY

Acute dystonia   sustained, often painful muscular spasms, producing twisting abnormal postures.

Acute Lymphoblastic Leukaemia (ALL)   a cancer of blood-forming cells in the bone marrow.

Adipose tissue   connective tissue consisting mainly of fat cells.

Adrenocorticotropin (ACTH)   a hormone produced by the pituitary gland, its key function is to stimulate the production and release of cortisol from the cortex of the adrenal gland.

Aetiology   the study of causation, or origination.

Agranulocytosis   an acute condition involving a severe and dangerous lowered white blood cell count.

Akathisa   a syndrome characterised by unpleasant sensations of inner restlessness that manifests itself with an inability to sit still or remain motionless.

Amenorrhoea   the absence of a menstrual period in a woman of reproductive age.

Amiodarone   a broad spectrum antiarrhythmic medication used to treat cardiac arrhythmias.

Anorgasmia   a type of sexual dysfunction in which a person cannot achieve orgasm.

Anticholinergic drugs   principally used for the treatment of drug-induced Parkinsonism, akathisia and acute dystonia; Parkinson disease; and Idiopathic or secondary dystonia. Examples include: procyclidine, oxybutinin and tolterodine.

Anticonvulsant medication   a diverse group of pharmaceuticals used in the treatment of epileptic seizures, increasingly being used as mood stabilisers in the treatment of bipolar disorder, examples include sodium valproate.

Antidepressant medication   drugs that relieve the symptoms of depression including amitriptyline, paroxetine, mirtazapine, lithium and venlafaxine.

Antipsychotic drugs   medication primarily used to manage psychosis (including delusions or hallucinations, as well as disordered thought), particularly in schizophrenia and bipolar disorder. A first generation of antipsychotics, known as typical antipsychotics, was discovered in the 1950s. Examples include: chlorpromazine, pimozide, mesoridazine, haloperidol, thioridazine and zuclopenthixol whilst second generation atypical antipsychotics, have been developed more recently, examples include: olanzapine, clozapine, aripiprazole, ziprasidone, quetiapine and risperidone.

Atheroma   fatty deposits in the walls of arteries.

Atherosclerosis   a hardening of the arteries caused by a build-up of fat, cholesterol, and other substances which collect in the walls of the arteries and form hard structures called plaques.

Avascular   having few or no blood vessels.

Benzodiazepines   a class of drugs with hypnotic, anxiolytic, anticonvulsive, amnestic and muscle relaxant properties. Often used to treat anxiety, sleeping problems and other disorders. Examples include: diazepam, lorazepam (trade name Ativan®), chlordiazepoxide, temazepam, nitrazepam, loprazolam and valium.

Bio-ethics   the study of controversial ethics brought about by advances in biology and medicine.

Blood dyscrasia   a diseased state of the blood, usually one in which the blood contains permanent abnormal cellular elements.

Bronchodilators   drugs which widen the air passages of the lungs and ease breathing by relaxing bronchial smooth muscle.

Candida albicans (thrush)   a colony of bacteria that grows in the intestinal tract of most adults. This can become a yeast infection if the healthy bacteria in the gastrointestinal tract become depleted.

Cardiac arrhythmia   a problem with the rate or rhythm of the heartbeat.

Cardiomyopathy   a weakening of the heart muscle or a change in the heart muscle.

Chemoreceptors   cells that respond to chemical stimuli.

Cholesterol   a waxy substance found in the body that is needed to produce hormones, vitamin D and bile.

Chronic bronchitis   a chronic inflammation of the bronchi (medium-size airways) in the lungs.

Chronic obstructive pulmonary disease (COPD)   the name for a collection of lung diseases including chronic bronchitis, emphysema and chronic obstructive airways disease.

Clostridium difficile   a type of bacteria found in the gut which does not usually cause problems in healthy people. However, when the healthy bacteria in the gut become depleted it can cause diarrhoea, nausea, and abdominal pain and can be life-threatening.

Collagen   a fibrous protein found in tissues such as tendon, ligament and skin.

Colonise   establish control over.

Conjunctivitis   a common infection of the conjunctiva which is the membrane covering the front of the eye.

Convulsions   a condition where body muscles contract and relax rapidly and repeatedly, resulting in an uncontrolled shaking of the body.

Corticosteroids   a group of steroid hormones with a wide range of physiological functions which are produced in the adrenal cortex or made synthetically.

Cortisol   a hormone released by the cortex of the adrenal gland and used to manage stress.

Creatine phosphokinase   an enzyme found mainly in the heart brain and skeletal muscle.

Cyanosis   the abnormal blue discoloration of the skin and mucous membranes, caused by a lack of oxygen in the blood.

Cytotoxic drugs   medication which is used to treat malignancies by directly killing tumour cells.

Decontamination   any activity that reduces the microbial load to prevent inadvertent contamination or infection.

Dermis   a layer of skin between the epidermis (with which it makes up the cutis) and subcutaneous tissues, that consists of connective tissue, supports the epidermis and cushions the body from stress and strain.

Diagnostic overshadowing   when a person's presenting symptoms are put down to their existing condition, rather than seeking another potentially treatable cause.

Diastolic   the time when the heart is in a period of relaxation, diastolic pressure is represented by the lower number in a blood pressure reading.

Disability adjusted life years (DALYs) a measure of overall disease burden, expressed as the number of years lost due to ill-health, disability or early death.

Dyslipidaemia an abnormal amount of lipids (e.g. cholesterol and/or fat) in the blood.

Electrocardiogram (ECG) a test that measures the electrical activity of the heart.

Emphysema a long-term, progressive disease of the lungs in which the alveoli are damaged causing shortness of breath.

Enteritis inflammation of the small intestine. Symptoms may include abdominal pain, diarrhoea, loss of appetite and vomiting.

Epidemiological the study of the distribution and patterns of health-events, health-characteristics and their causes or influences in well-defined populations.

Escherichia coli (E Coli) a bacterium commonly found in the lower intestine of warm-blooded organisms (endotherms). Most *E. coli* strains are harmless, but some types can cause serious food poisoning in humans.

Extrapyramidal symptoms (EPSES) a group of side effects such as parkinsonism, akathisia, dystonia, and tardive dyskinesia, commonly associated with antipsychotic medications.

Exudate any fluid that filters from the circulatory system into lesions or areas of inflammation.

Fibrinolysis a process that that occurs inside the body to break down blood clots.

Gangrene a serious and potentially life-threatening condition that arises when a considerable mass of body tissue dies (necrosis).

Glucometer a medical device for determining the approximate concentration of glucose in the blood.

Glycogen a polysaccharide that is the principal storage form of glucose (Glc) in animal and human cells.

Glycosuria the excretion of glucose into the urine.

Granulation tissue the perfused, fibrous connective tissue that replaces a fibrin clot in healing wounds.

Gynaecomastia   the abnormal development of large mammary glands in males resulting in breast enlargement.

Haemophilus influenza (flu)   a bacterial infection which can cause serious disease especially in young children.

Haemostasis   is a process which causes bleeding to stop.

Health care associated infections (HCAI)   infections that are acquired as a result of healthcare interventions.

Hemiparesis   weakness on one side of the body.

Herceptin   the brand name of a medicine called trastuzumab. It can stop the growth of breast cancer and sometimes reduce the size of the tumour.

Hirsutism   a condition with excess growth of hair in a male pattern caused by elevated levels of male sex hormones.

Histamine   a substance present in cells of the body which forms part of the immune response and is released when tissue is damaged and during an allergic reaction.

Homeostasis   the control of internal conditions, be it temperature, specific blood conditions or other variables within living organisms. Hypercholesterolemia high blood cholesterol levels.

Hyperglycaemia   a condition that occurs when your blood sugar (glucose) is too high.

Hyperprolactinaemia   the presence of abnormally-high levels of prolactin in the blood.

Hypoglycaemia   a condition that occurs when your blood sugar (glucose) is too low.

Hypotonic solution   a solution with a lower salt concentration than in the normal cells of the body and the blood.

Hypoxia   reduction of oxygen supply to a tissue below physiological levels despite adequate perfusion of the tissue by blood.

Idiosyncratic   an unusual feature of a person or object. The term is often used to express peculiarity.

Immunocompromised   susceptible to bacterial, fungal, and viral infections that healthy immune systems usually conquer.

Incretin injections a type of medication which works by increasing the levels of hormones called 'incretins'. These hormones help the body produce more insulin when needed and reduce the amount of glucose being produced by the liver.

Inherited mutations a genetic mutation that gets passed through the genes.

Ischemia a restriction in blood supply to tissues causing a shortage of oxygen and lucose needed for cellular metabolism.

Isotonic solution a solution that has the same salt concentration as the normal cells of the body and the blood.

Melanoma a cancerous condition of the melanocytic system of the skin and other organs.

Methicillin Resistant Staphylococcus Aureus (MRSA) strains of the bacteria, Staphylococcus aureus, that are resistant to a number of antibiotics, including methicillin.

Microbial load the number and type of micro-organisms contaminating an object.

Micro-organisms very tiny one-celled organisms, viruses, fungi, and bacteria.

Myalgia muscle pain or aching.

Myocardial infarction commonly referred to as a heart attack, is the death of heart uscle from the sudden blockage of a coronary artery by a blood clot.

Myocarditis an inflammation of the heart muscle.

Nebuliser a device used to administer medication in the form of a mist inhaled into the lungs.

Neutrophils the most common type of white blood cell.

Oculogyric crisis the name of a dystonic reaction to certain drugs or medical conditions.

Oedema a build-up of fluid in the tissues.

Oesophageal varices dilatated oesophageal veins often secondary to hypertension in the hepatic (liver) vessels.

Oestrogen the primary female sex hormones.

Opisthotonus   an inversely arching, hyperextension of the spine caused by spasm of the axial muscles along the spinal column.

Orthostatic hypotension   also called postural hypertension this is a form of hypotension in which a person's blood pressure suddenly falls when the person stands up or stretches.

Osteoporosis   a condition that affects the bones, causing them to become thin and weak.

Palliation   to treat it partially and insofar as possible, but not cure it completely.

Pathogens   an agent of disease.

Peak Expiratory Flow (PEF)   a person's maximum speed of expiration, as measured with a peak flow meter.

Pelvic inflammatory disease   an infection of the womb and/or fallopian tubes.

Platelet aggregation   the clumping together of platelets in the blood.

Polypharmacy   the use of multiple medications.

Proctitis   inflammation of the anus and rectum.

Progestogen   a group of female steroidal hormones including progesterone which is secreted by the ovaries as part of the menstrual cycle.

Prolactin   the hormone of lactation which is secreted by the pituitary gland.

Prophylactic   a preventive measure.

Purulent   containing, discharging, or causing the production of pus.

Pyrexia   fever of unknown origin in adults this is commonly defined as a temperature above 38.3 degrees celcius.

Reactive arthritis   also known as Reiter's syndrome, is a condition characterised by painful, swollen joints and is triggered by bacterial infection somewhere else in the body.

Repolarisation   the restoration of a polarised state across a membrane, as in a muscle fibre following contraction.

Serotonin   specific uptake inhibitors.

Serous fluid   any of various body fluids resembling serum which is typically pale yellow, transparent, and of a benign nature.

Systolic   the pressure exerted on the arterial walls by the blood when the ventricles of the heart contract, represented by the higher value in a blood pressure reading.

Tardive dystonia   abnormal tonicity of muscle, characterised by prolonged, repetitive muscle contractions that may cause twisting or jerking movements of the body or a body part.

Thrombocytopenia   an abnormal drop in the number of blood cells involved in forming blood clots.

Thrombotic   the formation or presence of a blood clot in a blood vessel.

Tuberculosis (TB)   a potentially fatal contagious disease caused by the bacterial micro-organism, tubercle bacillus or *Mycobacterium tuberculosis* that can affect almost any part of the body but is mainly an infection of the lungs.

Vasoconstriction   narrowing of the blood vessels resulting from contraction of the wall of the vessels.

Vasodilation   widening of blood vessels resulting from relaxation of the muscular wall of the vessels.

Viscosity   the quantity that describes a fluid's resistance to flow.

REFERENCES

Aboderin, I., Kalache, A., Ben-Shlomo, Y., Lynch, J.W., Yajnik, C.S., Kuh, D. and Yach, D. (2002) *Life Course Perspectives on Coronary Heart Disease, Stroke and Diabetes: Key Issues and Implications for Policy and Research*. Geneva: World Health Organization.

Adams, R.J., Wilson, D.H., Taylor, A.W., Daly, A., Tursan d'Espaignet, E., Dal Grande, E. and Ruffin, R.E. (2004) Psychological factors and asthma quality of life: a population based study. *Thorax*, 59: 930–35.

Adamson Greene, C.F. and Rosen, J.A. (2008) Psychotropic medications and metabolic disorders. In A.R. Rosen and D.A. Wirshing (eds), *Diabetes and the Metabolic Syndrome in Mental Health*. Philadelphia, PA: Wolters Kluwer and Lippincott Williams & Wilkins.

Adler, M. (2004) Why sexually transmitted infections are important. In M. Adler, F. Cowan, P. French, H. Mitchell and J. Richens (eds), *ABC of Sexually Transmitted Infections*, 5th edn. London: BMJ Books.

Adnet, P., Lestavel P. and Krivosic-Horber, R. (2000) Neuroleptic malignant syndrome. *British Journal of Anaesthesia*, 85: 129–35.

Alberti, K.G.M.M., Kimmet, P. and Shaw, J. (2006) Metabolic syndrome – a new world-wide definition: a consensus statement from the International Diabetes Federation. *Diabetic Medicine*, 23: 469–80.

Alcohol Concern (2010) *Factsheet: The Impact of Alcohol on Health*. London: Alcohol Concern.

Allison, D.B., Newcomer, J.W., Dunn, A.L., Blumenthal, J.A., Fabricatore, A.N., Daumit, G.L., Cope, M.B., Riley, W.T., Vreeland, B., Hibbeln, J.R. and Alpert, J.E. (2009) Obesity among those with mental disorders: a National Institute of Mental Health meeting report. *American Journal of Preventive Medicine*, 36(4): 341–50.

Almeida, C.A. and Barry, S.A. (2010) *Cancer: Basic Science and Clinical Aspects*. Chichester, UK: Wiley-Blackwell.

Andersohn, F., Schade, R., Suissa, S. and Garbe, E. (2009) Long-term use of antidepressants for depressive disorders and the risk of diabetes mellitus. *American Journal of Psychiatry*, 166(5): 591–8.

Angeras, M., Brandberg, A., Falk, A. and Seeman, T. (1992) Comparison between sterile saline and tap water for the cleaning of acute traumatic soft tissue wounds. *European Journal of Surgery*, 158: 347–50.

Aronoff, S.L., Bertowitz, K., Shreine, B. and Want, L. (2004) Glucose metabolism and regulation: beyond insulin and glucagon. *Diabetes Spectrum*, 17(3): 183–90.

Ashcroft, J. (2011) The importance of physical health assessment. In D.B. Cooper (ed.), *Introduction to Mental Health: Substance Use*. Oxford: Radcliffe Press.

Ashton, M., Miller, C.L., Bowden, J.A. and Bertossa, S. (2010) People with mental illness can tackle tobacco. *Australian and New Zealand Journal of Psychiatry*, 44: 1021–8.

Asthma UK (2011) *All About Asthma*. London: Asthma UK.

Atakan, Z. (2008) Cannabis use by people with severe mental illness – is it important? *Advances in Psychiatric Treatment*, 14: 423–31.

Audrain-McGovern, J., Lerman, C., Wileyto, E.P., Rodriguez, D. and Shields, P.G. (2004) Interacting effects of genetic predisposition and depression on adolescent smoking progression. *American Journal of Psychiatry*, 161: 1224–30.

Azadbakht, L., Mirmiran, P., Esmaillzadeh, A., Azizi, T. and Azizi, F. (2005) Beneficial effects of a dietary approaches to stop hypertension eating plan on features of the metabolic syndrome. *Diabetes Care*, 28: 2823–31.

Babić, D., Maslov, B., Martinac, M., Nikolić, K., Uzun, S. and Kozumplik, O. (2010) Bipolar disorder and metabolic syndrome: comorbidity or side effects of treatment of bipolar disorder. *Psychiatr Danub*, 22: 75–8.

Baid, H. (2006) The process of conducting a physical assessment: a nursing perspective. *British Journal of Nursing*, 15(13): 710–14.

Bale, S. and Jones, V. (2006) *Wound Care Nursing: A Patient Centred Approach*. Edinburgh: Mosby.

Ballon, J.A. and Fernandez, J.W. (2008) Diabetes and mental health. In A.R. Rosen and D.A. Wirshing (eds), *Diabetes and the Metabolic Syndrome in Mental Health*. Philadelphia, PA: Wolters Kluwer and Lippincott Williams & Wilkins.

Bandura, A. (2000) Health promotion from the perspective of social cognition theory. In P. Norman, C. Abraham and M. Conner (eds), *Understanding and Changing Health Behaviour – from Health Beliefs to Self-Regulation*. Amsterdam: Harwood Academic Publishers.

Bandura, A. (2002) Self-efficacy assessment. In R. Fernandez-Ballesteros (ed.), *Encyclopedia of Psychological Assessment*. London: Sage.

Banham, L. and Gilbody, S. (2010) Smoking cessation in severe mental illness: what works? *Addiction*, 105: 1176–89.

Bannerman, M. and Proom, T. (2009) Sexually acquired infections. In K. French (ed.), *Sexual Health*. Oxford: Wiley-Blackwell.

Baranowski, T., Perry, C. L. and Parcel, G.S. (2002) How individuals, environments, and health behaviour interact – social cognitive theory. In K. Glanz, B.K. Rimer and F.M. Lewis (eds), *Health Behaviour and Health Education: Theory, Research and Practice*, 3rd edn. San Francisco: Jossey-Bass.

Barber, P., Brown, R. and Martin, D. (2009a) *Mental Health Law in England and Wales: A Guide for Mental Health Professionals*. Exeter: Learning Matters Ltd.

Barber, P., Brown, R. and Martin, D. (2009b) *The Mental Capacity Act 2005: A Guide for Practice*, 2nd edn. Exeter: Learning Matters Ltd.

Barre, L.K., Ferron, J.C., Davis, K.E. and Whitley, R. (2011) Healthy eating in persons with serious mental illnesses: understanding and barriers. *Psychiatric Rehabilitation Journal*, 34(4): 304–10.

Bazire, S. (2007) *Psychotropic Drug Directory 2007: The Professionals' Pocket Handbook – an Aide-Mémoire*. Trowbridge, UK: Cromwell Press.

Bekaert, S. and White, A. (2006) *Integrated Contraceptive and Sexual Healthcare: A Practical Guide*. Oxford: Radcliffe Press.

Benbow, M. and Deacon, M. (2011) Helping people who self-harm to care for their wounds. *Mental Health Practice*, 14(6): 28–31.

Bennett, G., Dealey, C. and Possnett, J. (2004) The cost of pressure ulcers in the UK. *Age and Ageing*, 33: 230–35.

Berkman, L.F. and Kawachi, I. (eds) (2000) *Social Epidemiology*. Oxford: Oxford University Press.

BHF (2008a) *European Cardiovascular Disease Statistics: 2008 Edition*. Oxford: British Heart Foundation Health Promotion Research Group and the Health Economics Research Group.

BHF (2008b) *Coronary Heart Disease Statistics: 2008 Edition*. Oxford: British Heart Foundation Health Promotion Research Group.

Blair, I. (2009) Infection prevention and control in the community. In A.P. Fraise and C.R. Bradley (eds), *Ayliffe's Control of Healthcare-Associated Infection*, 5th edn. London: Hodder Arnold.

Blunt, J. (2001) Wound cleansing: ritualistic or research-based practice? *Nursing Standard*, 16(1): 33–6.

Blythe, J. and White, J. (2012) Role of the mental health nurse towards physical health care in serious mental illness: an integrative review of 10 years of UK literature. *International Journal of Mental Health Nursing*, 21: 193–201.

Bobes, J., Arango, C., Garcia-Garcia, M. and Rejas, J. (2010) Healthy lifestyle habits and 10-year cardiovascular risk in schizophrenia spectrum disorders: an analysis of the impact of smoking tobacco in the CLAMORS schizophrenia cohort. *Schizophrenia Research*, 119: 101–9.

Bowell, B. (1992) Protecting the patient at risk. *Nursing Times*, 88(3): 32–5.

Boyajian, R. (2010) Depressions impact on survival in patients with cancer. *Clinical Journal of Oncology Nursing*, 14(5): 549–652.

Bradshaw, T., Lovell, K. and Campbell, M. (2010) The development and evaluation of a complex health education intervention for adults with a diagnosis of schizophrenia. *Journal of Psychiatric and Mental Health Nursing*, 17: 473–86.

Bradshaw, T., Lovell, K. and Harris, N. (2005) Healthy living interventions and schizophrenia: a systematic review. *Journal of Advanced Nursing*, 49(6): 634–654.

Bradshaw, T. and Pedley, R. (2012) Evolving role of mental health nurses in the physical health care of people with serious mental health illness. *International Journal of Mental Health Nursing*, 21: 266–73.

Bridgewater, J. and Gore, M. (2008) Developments in cancer treatment. In Corner, J. and Bailey, C. (eds) *Cancer Nursing. Care in Context*. Second edition. Oxford: Blackwell.

British Formulary Committee (2010) *British National Formulary 60*. London: British Medical Association and Pharmaceutical Press.

British Formulary Committee (2011) *British National Formulary*. London: British Medical Association and Royal Pharmaceutical Society.

British Thoracic Society (2006) *The Burden of Lung Disease Reports*. London: BMJ.

Brock, D.W. (2007) Patient competence and surrogate decision-making. In R. Rhodes, L.P. Francis and A. Silvers (eds), *The Blackwell Guide to Medical Ethics*. Oxford: Blackwell.

Brown, S. and Smith, E. (2009) Can a brief health promotion intervention delivered by mental health keyworkers improve clients' physical health: a randomized control trial. *Journal of Mental Health*, 18: 372–8.

Brown, A., Yung, A., Cosgrove, E., Killackey, E., Buckby, J. et al. (2006) Depressed mood as a risk factor for unprotected sex in young people. *Australian Psychiatry*, 14(3): 310–12.

Brown, A.P., Lubman, D.I. and Paxton, S.J. (2008) STIs and blood-borne viruses: risk factors for individuals with mental illness. *Australian Family Physician*, 37(7): 531–4.

Brown, C., Leith, J., Dickerson, F., Medoff, D., Kreyenbuhl, J., Fang, L., Goldberg, R., Potts, W. and Dixon, L. (2010) Predictors of mortality in patients with serious mental illness and co-occurring type 2 diabetes. *Psychiatry Research*, 177: 250–54.

Brown, S. (1997) Excess mortality of schizophrenia: a meta-analysis. *British Journal of Psychiatry*, 154: 672–6.

Brown, S., Birtwistle, J., Roe, L. and Thompson, C. (1999) The unhealthy lifestyle of people with schizophrenia. *Psychological Medicine*, 29: 697–701.

Brown, S., Inskip, H. and Barraclough, B. (2000) Causes of the excess mortality of schizophrenia. *British Journal of Psychiatry*, 177: 121–217.

Brown, S., Kim, M., Mitchell, C. and Inskip, H. (2010) Twenty-five year mortality of a community cohort with schizophrenia. *British Journal of Psychiatry*, 196: 116–21.

Buck, A., Blackhall, A. and Wood S (2009) The mental health of older adults. In N. Wycraft (ed.) *An Introduction to Mental Health Nursing*. Maridenhead: McGraw Hill, 143–156.

Burrows, G. (2011) Lesbian, bisexual and transgender health. *Practice Nurse*, 41(3): 23–5.

Bushe, C., Yeomans, D., Floyd, T. and Smith, S.M. (2008) Categorical prevalence and severity of hyperprolactinaemia in two UK cohorts of patients with severe mental illness during
treatment with antipsychotics. *Journal of Psychopharmacology*, 22(2): 56–6.

Cabassa, L.J., Ezell, J.M. and Lewis-Fernandez, R. (2010) Lifestyle interventions for adults with
serious mental illness: a systematic literature review. *Psychiatric Services*, 61(8): 774–82.

Care Quality Commission (2008) *Registering with the Care Quality Commission in Relation
to Healthcare-Associated Infection: Guidance for Trust 2009/10.* London: CQC.

Care Quality Commission (2011) *Community Mental Health Services Survey 2011.* London:
CQC. Available at: www.nhssurveys.org (accessed 16 September 2012).

Carey, M.P., Ravi, V., Prabha, S., Chandra, S., Desai, A. and Neal, D.J. (2007) Prevalence
of HIV, hepatitis B, syphilis and chlamydia among adults seeking treatment for a mental
health disorder in Southern India. *AIDS Behaviour*, 11: 289–97.

Carmena, R. (2003) The metabolic syndrome. *Archives of International Medicine*, 163:
427–36.

Casagrande, S.S., Jerome, G.J., Dalcin, A.T., Dickerson, F.B., Anderson, C.A., Appel, L.J.,
Charleston, J., Crum, R.M., Young, D.R., Guallar, E., Frick, K.D., Goldberg, R.W., Oefin-
ger, M., Finkelstein,J., Gennusa III J.V., Fred-Omojole, O., Campbell, L.M., Wang,
N.-Y. and Daumit, G.L. (2010) Randomized trial of achieving healthy lifestyles in psychiatric rehabilitation: the ACHIEVE trial. *BMC Psychiatry*, 10: 108 (www.biomedcentral.
com/1471-244X/10/108, 18 July 2012).

Catts, V.S., Catts, S.V., O'Toole, B.I. and Frost, A.D. (2008) Cancer incidence in patients with
schizophrenia and their first-degree relatives – a meta-analysis. *Acta Psychiatrica Scandinavica*, 117: 323–36.

Chadwick, A., Street, S., McAndrew, S. and Deacon, M. (2012) Minding our own bodies:
reviewing the literature regarding the perceptions of service users diagnosed with serious
mental illness on barriers to accessing physical health care. *International Journal of Mental
Health Nursing*, 21: 211–19.

Chafetz, L., White, M., Collins-Bride, G., Cooper, B.A. and Nickens, J. (2008) Clinical trial of
wellness training health promotion for severely mentally ill adults. *The Journal of Nervous
and Mental Disease*, 196(6): 475–83.

Cheng, V.C.C., Wu, A.K.L., Cheung, C.H.Y., Lau, S.K.P., Woo, P.C.Y., Chan, K.H., Li, K.S.M.,
Ip, I.K.S., Dunn, E.L.W. and Lee, R.A. et al. (2007) Outbreak of human metapneumovirus
infection in psychiatric inpatients: implications for directly observed use of alcohol hand rub
in prevention of nosocomial outbreaks. *Journal of Hospital Infection*, 67: 336–43.

Colagiuri, S., Foster-Powell, K. and Brand Miller, J. (1997) *The Pocket Guide to the Glucose
Revolution for People with Diabetes.* London: Hodder & Stoughton.

Collier, M. (2002) Wound bed preparation. *Nursing Times*, 98(2): 55–7 (NT Plus Wound
Care Supplement).

Collier, M. (2004) Recognition and management of wound infections. Retrieved from: www.
worldwidewounds.com/2004/january/Collier/Management-of-Wound-infections.html
(accessed 1 May 2012).

Cooper, P. and Evans, J. (2007) Collaborative working: tackling violence, aggression and dual
diagnosis. *Mental Health Nursing*, 27(2): 16–19.

Cunliffe, J. and Fawcett, I. (2002) Wound cleansing: the evidence for the techniques and solutions used. *Professional Nurse*, 18(2): 95–9.

Cutting, K. and Harding, K. (1994) Criteria for identifying wound infection. *Journal of
Wound Care*, 3(4): 198–201.

Cuzzell, J.Z. (1988) Woundcare forum the New Ryb Color code. *American Journal of Nursing*, 88(10): 1342–6.

Daniels, L. (2002) Diet and coronary heart disease. *Nursing Standard*, 16(43): 47–54.

Davis, M.F., Shapiro, D., Windsor, R., Whalen, P., Rhode, R., Miller, H.S. and Sechrest, L. (2011) Motivational interviewing versus prescriptive advice for smokers who are ready to quit. *Patient Education and Counselling*, 83: 129–33.

Day, J.C., Wood, G., Dewey, M. and Bentall, R.P. (1995) A self rating scale for measuring neuroleptic side effects: validation in a group of schizophrenic patients. *British Journal of Psychiatry*, 166(5): 650–53.

Deakin, T. (2011) *X-PERT Audit Report: X-PERT National Results Organizations Comparisons. How Are You Doing?* Hebden Bridge, Yorkshire: X-PERT Community Interest Company.

Dealey C. (2005) *The Care of Wounds: A Guide for Nurses*. Oxford: Blackwell Science.

Dealey, C. and Cameron, J. (2008) *Wound Management*. Oxford: Wiley-Blackwell.

Dean, J., Todd, G. and Morrow, H. (2001) Mum I used to be good looking … look at me now: the physical health needs of adults with mental health problems. *International Journal of Health Promotion*, 3: 16–24.

De Hert, M., Schreurs, V., Vancampfort, D. and van Winkel, R. (2009) Metabolic syndrome in people with schizophrenia: a review. *World Psychiatry*, 8: 15–22.

De Leon, J., Becona, E., Gurpegui, M., Gonzalez-Pinto, A. and Diaz, F.J. (2002) The association between high nicotine dependence and severe mental illness may be consistent across countries. *Journal of Clinical Psychiatry*, 63(9): 812–16.

Department of Health (1995) *HSG (95)18: Hospital laundry arrangements for used and infected linen*. London: Department of Health.

Department of Health (1999) *National Service Framework for Mental Health*. London: Department of Health.

Department of Health (2000) *National Service Framework for Coronary Heart Disease*. London: Department of Health.

Department of Health (2001) *National Strategy for Sexual Health and HIV*. London: Department of Health.

Department of Health (2002) *Mental Health Policy Implementation Guidelines: Dual Diagnosis Good Practice Guide*. London: Department of Health.

Department of Health (2003) *Delivering Investment in General Practice: Implementing the New GMS Contract*. London: Department of Health.

Department of Health (2004a) *Choosing Health: Making Healthier Choices*. London: Department of Health.

Department of Health (2004b) *Towards Cleaner Hospitals and Lower Rates of Infection*. London: Department of Health.

Department of Health (2005a) *The Mental Capacity Act 2005*. London: HMSO.

Department of Health (2005b) *Meeting the Physical Needs of Individuals with Mental Health Problems and the Mental Health Needs of Individuals Cared for in General Health Sectors: Advice from the Standing Nursing and Midwifery Advisory Committee*. London: Department of Health.

Department of Health (2005c) *Mental Capacity Act 2005 Code of Practice*. London: Department of Health.

Department of Health (2006a) *Choosing Health: Supporting the Physical Health Needs of People with Severe Mental Illness*. Commissioning Framework. London: Department of Health.

Department of Health (2006b) *From Values to Action: The Chief Nursing Officer's Review of Mental Health Nursing*. London: Department of Health.

Department of Health (2006c) *Dual Diagnosis in Mental Health Inpatient and Day Hospital Settings*. London: Department of Health.

Department of Health (2006d) *Saving Lives: A Delivery Programme to Reduce Healthcare Associated Infection, including MRSA Screening for Meticillin-resistant Staphylococcus*

Aureus (MRSA) Colonisation: A Strategy for NHS Trusts: A Summary of Best Practice. London: Department of Health.

Department of Health (2007) *The Mental Health Act 2007*. London: HMSO.

Department of Health (2008) *Clean, Safe Care: Reducing Infections and Saving Lives*. London: Department of Health.

Department of Health (2009a) *New Horizons: A Shared Vision for Mental Health*. London: Department of Health.

Department of Health (2009b) *A Guide for the Management of Dual Diagnosis in Prisons*. London: Department of Health.

Department of Health (2009c) *The Health and Social Care Act 2008: Code of Practice for the NHS on the Prevention and Control of Health Care Associated Infections and Related Guidance*. London: Department of Health.

Department of Health (2010) *Uniform and Workwear: Guidance on Uniform and Workwear Policies for NHS Employers*. London: Department of Health.

Department of Health (2011a) *No Health without Mental Health: A Cross-government Mental Health Outcomes Strategy for People of All Ages*. London: Department of Health.

Department of Health (2011b) *Improving Outcomes: A Strategy for Cancer*. London: Department of Health (available at: www.dh.gov.uk).

Department of Health (2011c) *Patient-centred NHS a Step Closer to Reality* (Health and Social Care Bill). London: Department of Health.

Department of Health (2011d) *Safe Management of Healthcare Waste*. London: Department of Health.

Diabetes UK (2009) *Prediabetes: Preventing the Type 2 Diabetes Epidemic*. London: Diabetes UK.

Diabetes UK (2011a) *Ketoacidosis (DKA): The Balance Guide to All the Diabetes Meters, Medications, Insulins, Pens and Pumps Available in the UK, 2011–2012*. London: Diabetes UK.

Diabetes UK (2011b) *Evidence-based Nutrition Guidelines for the Prevention and Management of Diabetes*. London: Diabetes UK. Available at: www.diabetes.org.uk/nutrition-guidelines (accessed 18 July 2012).

DiClemente, C.C., Delahanty, J.C., Kofeldt, M.G., Dixon, L., Goldberg, R. and Lucksted, A. (2011) Stage movement following a 5As intervention in tobacco dependent individuals with serious mental illness (SMI). *Addictive Behaviours*, 36: 261–4.

Dimond, B. (2008) *Legal Aspects of Mental Capacity*, 2nd edn. Oxford: Wiley-Blackwell.

Disability Rights Commission (2006) *Equal Treatment: Closing the Gap*. Stratford upon Avon: Disability Rights Commission.

Disability Rights Commission (2007) *Equal Treatment: Closing the Gap One Year On*. Stratford upon Avon: Disability Rights Commission.

Dougherty, L. and Bailey, C. (2008) Chemotherapy. In J. Corner and C. Bailey (eds), *Cancer Nursing: Care in Context*, 2nd edn. Oxford: Blackwell.

Dougherty, L. and Lister, S. (2011) *Royal Marsden Hospital Manual of Clinical Nursing Procedures*. London: Wiley-Blackwell.

Drake, R.E. and Wallach, M.A. (2000) Dual diagnosis: 15 years of progress. *Psychiatric Services*, 51(9): 1126–9.

Drake, R.E., Wallach, M.A., Teague, G.B., Freeman, D. H., Paskus, T.S. and Clark, T.A. (1991) Housing instability and homelessness among rural schizophrenic patients. *American Journal of Psychiatry*, 148: 330–36.

Editorial (2011) No mental health without physical health. *The Lancet*, 377: 611.

Eldridge, D., Dawber, N. and Gray, R. (2011) A well-being support program for patients with severe mental illness: a service evaluation. *BMC Psychiatry*, 11(46).

Esposito, K., Marfella, R., Ciotola, M., Di Palo, C., Giugliano, F., Giugliano, G., D'Armiento, M., D'Andrea, F. and Giugliano, D. (2004) Effect of Mediterranean-style diet on endothelial dysfunction and markers of vascular inflammation in the metabolic syndrome: a randomized trial. *JAMA*, 292: 144–6.

Epstein, O., Perkin, G.D., Cookson, J. and de Bono, D.P. (2003) *Clinical Examination*, 3rd edn. Edinburgh: Mosby.

European Monitoring Centre for Drugs and Drug Addiction (2010) *Annual Report 2010: The State of the Drugs Problem in Europe*. Luxemburg: European Monitoring Centre for Drugs and Drug Addiction.

European Pressure Ulcer Advisory Panel (2009) *Prevention of Pressure Ulcers: Quick Reference Guide*. Available at: www.epuap.org/guidelines/Final_Quick_Prevention.pdf (accessed 5 May 2012).

European Wound Management Association (2006) *Position Document: Management of wound infection*. Available at: http://ewma.org/fileadmin/user_upload/EWMA/pdf/Position_Documents/2006/English_ps_doc_2006.pdf (accessed 7 July 2012).

Ewles, L. and Simnett, I. (2003) *Promoting Health: A Practical Guide to Health Education*, 5th edn. London: Bailliere Tindall.

Faithfull, S. (2008) Radiotherapy. In J. Corner and C. Bailey (eds), *Cancer Nursing: Care in Context*, 2nd edn. Oxford: Blackwell.

Farr, S.L., Curtis, K.M., Robbins, C.L., Zapata, L.B. and Dietz, P.M. (2010) Use of contraception among US women with frequent mental distress. *Contraception*, 83: 127–33.

Faulkner, G., Cohn, T. and Remington, G. (2010) Interventions to reduce weight gain in schizophrenia (review). *The Cochrane Library*, Issue 3. The Cochrane Collaboration, published by John Wiley &Sons, Ltd.

Faulkner, G., Taylor, A., Munro, S., Selby, P. and Gee, C. (2007) The acceptability of physical activity programming within a smoking cessation service for individuals with severe mental illness. *Patient Education and Counseling*, 66: 123–6.

Fernandez, R., Griffiths, R. and Ussia, C. (2002) Water for wound cleansing. *The Cochrane Database of Systematic Reviews*. Issue 4: art no. cd 003861. The Cochrane Collaboration, published by John Wiley &Sons, Ltd.

Fettes, A.M. (2006) A clinimetric analysis of wound management tools. Available at: www.worldwidewounds.com/2006/January/Fettes/clinimetric-Analysis-wound-Measurement-tools.html (accessed April 2012).

Field, G.C., Simpson, K.W. and Bond, E.F. (2004) Clinical nurse specialists and nurse practitioners: complementary roles for infectious disease and infection control. *American Journal of Infection Control*, 32(4): 239–42.

Filik, R., Sipos, F.R., Kehoe, P.G., Burns, T., Cooper, S.J., Stevens, H., Laugharne, R., Young, G., Perrington, S., McKendrick, J., Stevenson, D. and Harrison, G. (2006) The cardiovascular and respiratory health of people with schizophrenia. *Acta Psychiatrica Scandinavica*, 113: 298–305.

Flanagan, M. (1997) *Wound Management*. London: Churchill Livingstone.

Fraise, A.P. and Bradley, C.R. (eds) (2009) *Ayliffe's Control of Healthcare-Associated Infection*, 5th edn. London: Hodder Arnold.

Francis, L.P. (2007) Discrimination in medical practice: Justice and the obligations of health care providers to disadvantaged patients. In R. Rhodes, L.P. Francis and A. Silvers (eds), *The Blackwell Guide to Medical Ethics*. Oxford: Blackwell.

French, K. (2009) Contraception including emergency contraception. In K. French (ed.), *Sexual Health*. Oxford: Wiley-Blackwell.

Friedli, L. and Dardis, C. (2002) Smoke gets in their eyes. *Mental Health Today*, January: 18–21.

Galletly, C.L. and Murray, L.E. (2009) Managing weight in persons living with severe mental illness in community settings: a review of strategies used in community interventions. *Issues in Mental Health Nursing*, 30: 660–68.

Gallo-Silver, L. and Weiner, M.O. (2006) Survivors of sexual abuse diagnosed with cancer: managing the impact of early trauma on cancer. *Journal of Psychosocial Oncology*, 24 (1): 107–134.

Garden, G. (2005) Physical examination in psychiatric practice. *Advances in Psychiatric Treatment*, 11: 142–9.

Gibody, S. (2010) *Smoking Cessation for People with Severe Mental Illness: A Pilot Sudy and Definitive Randomised Evaluation of a Bespoke Service*. NIHR Health Technology Assessment Programme. Available at: www.hta.ac.uk/project/1839.asp (accessed 15 July 2012).

Glasier, A. and Gebbie, A. (2008) *Handbook of Family Planning and Reproductive Healthcare*, 5th edn. Edinburgh: Churchill Livingstone Elsevier.

Glassman, A.H. and Bigger, J.T. (2001) Antipsychotic drugs: prolonged QTc interval, Torsade de Pointes, and sudden death. *American Journal of Psychiatry*, 158: 1774–82.

Gold Standards Framework Centre (2010) *Overview of the Gold Standards Framework Centre*. Available at: www.goldstandardsframework.org.uk (accessed 17 May 2012).

Goldman, L.S. (1999) Medical illness in patients with schizophrenia. *Journal of Clinical Psychiatry*, 60(21): 10–15.

Gooptu, B., Ward, L., Ansari, A.O., Eraut, C.D., Law, D. and Davidson, A.G. (2006) Oxygen alert cards and controlled oxygen: preventing emergency admissions at risk of hypercapnic acidosis receiving high inspired oxygen concentrations in ambulances and A&E departments. *Emergency Medicine Journal*, 23: 636–8.

Gorczynski, P. and Faulkner, G. (2010) Exercise therapy for schizophrenia (review). *The Cochrane Library*, Issue 6. The Cochrane Collaboration, published by John Wiley & Sons, Ltd.

Gough, S. and Peveler, R. (2004) Diabetes and its prevention: pragmatic solutions for people with schizophrenia. *British Journal of Psychiatry*, 184(47): 106–11.

Goulet, K. and Grignon, S. (2008) Case report: clozapine given in the context of chemotherapy for lung cancer. *Psycho-oncology*, 17(5): 512–6.

Gray, R. (2012) Physical health and mental illness: a silent scandal. *International Journal of Mental Health Nursing*, 21: 191–2.

Gray, R., Hardy, S. and Anderson, K.H. (2009) Physical health and severe mental illness: If we don't do something about it, who will? *International Journal of Mental Health Nursing*, 18: 299–300.

Gray, R., Parr, A.M. and Robson, D. (2005) Has tardive dyskinesia disappeared? *Mental Health Practice*, 8(10): 20–22.

Green, B. (2004) *Focus on Antipsychotics*. Newbury, UK: Petroc Press.

Green, B. (2009) The decline of NHS inpatient psychiatry in England. Available at: http://priory.com/psychiatry/Decline_NHS_Inpatient_Psychiatry.htm (accessed 6 January 2012).

Gregory, R.L. (2004) *Oxford Companion to the Mind*, 2nd edn. Oxford: Oxford University Press.

Griffiths, M., Kidd, S.A., Pike, S. and Chan, J. (2010) The Tobacco Addiction Recovery Program: initial outcome findings. *Archives of Psychiatric Nursing*, 24(4): 239–46.

Griffiths, R., Fernandez, R. and Ussia, C. (2001) Is tap water a safe alternative to normal saline for wound irrigation in the community setting? *Journal of Wound Care*, 10(10): 407–10.

Grose, S. and Schub, T. (2010) Quick lesson about tuberculosis: adult. *Cinahl Information systems*. California.

Grundy, S.M. (2005) Metabolic Syndrome scientific statement by the American Heart Association and the National Heart, Lung and Blood Institute, *Arterioscl Thromb Vas Biol*; 24: 2243–2244.

Guillebaud, J. and Macgregor, A. (2009) *The Pill and Other Forms of Hormonal Contraception*, 7th edn. New York: Oxford University Press.

Gunnewicht, B. and Dunford, C. (2004) *Fundamental Aspects of Tissue Viability Nursing*. Salisbury: Quay Books.

Hamer, S. and Haddad, P. (2007) Adverse effects of antipsychotics as outcome measures. *British Journal of Psychiatry*, 191: 50.

Hamera, E., Goetz, J., Brown, C. and Van Sciver, A. (2010) Safety considerations when promoting exercise in individuals with serious mental illness. *Psychiatry Research*, 178: 220–22.

Happell, B., Davies, C. and Scott, D. (2012a) Health behavior interventions to improve physical health in individuals diagnosed with a mental illness: a systematic review. *International Journal of Mental Health Nursing*, 21: 236–47.

Happell, B., Scott, D., Platania-Phung, C. and Nankivell, J. (2012b) Should we or shouldn't we? Mental Health Nurses' views on physical health care of mental health consumers. *International Journal of Mental Health Nursing*, 21: 202–10.

Hardy, S. and Thomas, B. (2012) Mental and physical health comorbidity: political imperatives and practice implications. *International Journal of Mental Health Nursing*, 21: 289–98.

Harris, C.E. and Barraclough, B. (1998) Excess mortality of mental disorder. *British Journal of Psychiatry*, 173: 11–53.

Havard, D. and Western, C. (2007) A snapshot of England's tissue viability services. *Wounds UK*, 3(2): 13–19.

Hassapidou, M., Papadimitriou, K., Athanasiadou, N., Tokmakidou, V., Pagkalos, I., Vlahavas, G. and Tsofliou, F. (2011) Changes in body weight, body composition and cardiovascular risk factors after long-term nutritional intervention in patients with severe mental illness: an observational study. *BMC Psychiatry*, 11: 31

Hawton, K., Bale, L., Casey, D., Shepherd, A., Simkin, S. and Harris, L. (2006) Monitoring deliberate self-harm presentations to general hospitals. *Crisis*, 27(4): 157–63.

Health and Safety Executive (1992) *The Personal Protective Equipment at Work Regulations: Guidance on Regulations*. London: The Stationery Office.

Health and Social Care Information Centre (2011) *Mental Capacity Act 2005: Deprivation of Liberty Safeguards Assessments (England)*. Second report on annual data 2010/11. London: HSCIC. Available at: www.ic.nhs.uk (accessed 17 April 2012).

Healthcare Commission (2008) *The Pathway to Recovery*. London: Healthcare Commission.

Healy, D. (2009) *Psychiatric Drugs Explained*, 5th edn. London: Elsevier.

Heatherton, T.F., Kozlowski, L.T., Frecker, R.C. and Fagerström, K.O. (1991) The Fagerström Test for Nicotine Dependence: a revision of the Fagerström Tolerance Questionnaire. *British Journal of Addiction*, 86: 1119–27.

Hennekens, C.H., Hennekens, A.R., Hollar, D. and Casey, D.E. (2005) Schizophrenia and increased risks of cardiovascular disease. *American Heart Journal*, 150(6): 1115–21.

Higgins, A., Barker, P. and Begley, C. (2006) Sexual health education for people with mental health problems: what can we learn from the literature? *Journal of Psychiatric and Mental Health Nursing*, 13: 687–97.

Hilton, S., Hunt, K., Emslie, C., Salinas, M. and Ziebland, S. (2008) Have men been overlooked? A comparison of young men and women's experiences of chemotherapy-induced alopecia. *Psycho-Oncology*, 17: 577–583.

Himelhoch, S., Lehman, A., Kreyenbuhl, J., Daumit, G.M.D., Brown, C. and Dixon, L. (2004) Prevalence of chronic obstructive pulmonary disease among those with serious mental illness. *American Journal of Psychiatry*, 161: 2317–19.

Hippisley-Cox, J., Parker, C., Coupland, C. and Vinogradova, Y. (2007) Inequalities in the primary care of patients with coronary heart disease and serious mental illness: a cross sectional study. *Heart*, 93(10): 1256–62.

Hodgson, R. and Adeyemo, O. (2004) Physical examination performed by psychiatrists. *International Journal of Psychiatry in Clinical Practice*, 8(1): 57–60.

Hoffman, P. (2009) Laundry, kitchens and healthcare waste. In A.P. Fraise and C.R. Bradley (eds), *Ayliffe's Control of Healthcare-Associated Infection*, 5th edn. London: Hodder Arnold.

Holt, R.I.G. (2010) The weight of the world: the burden and management of antipsychotic induced obesity (23rd ECNP Congress – Tuesday 31 August 2010), *European Neuropsychopharmacology*, 20(3) (Suppl.): S195.

Holt, R.I.G. and Peveler, R.C. (2006) Association between antipsychotic drugs and diabetes. *Diabetes, Obesity and Metabolism*, 8: 125–35.

Horrocks, J., Price, S., House, A. and Owens, D. (2003) Self-injury attendances in the accident and emergency department: clinical database study. *British Journal of Psychiatry*, 183: 34–9.

Hospital Infection Society (2006) *Preliminary Results of Third Prevalence Survey of HCAI in England 2006 – Report for Department of Health*. London: Hospital Infection Society.

Howard, L. and Gamble, C. (2011) Supporting mental health nurses to address the physical health needs of people with serious mental illness in acute inpatient care settings. *Journal of Psychiatric and Mental Health Nursing*, 18: 105–12.

Howard, L.M., Barley, E.A., Davies, E., Rigg, A., Lempp, H., Rose, D., Taylor, D. and Thornicroft, G. (2010) Cancer diagnosis in people with severe mental illness: practical and ethical issues. *Lancet Oncology*, 11: 797–804.

Hughes, J. (2011) An ethnographic study of infection prevention and control practices in a mental health trust. Salford Postgraduate Annual Research Conference (SPARC), University of Salford, Manchester, June.

Hughes, J., Blackman, H., McDonald, E., Hull, S. and Fitzpatrick, B. (2011a) Involving service users in infection control practice. *Nursing Times*, 7(25): 18–19.

Hughes, J., Jennings, L. and Rosbottom, L. (2010) Infection prevention and control in mental health: different bugs or different approaches? (Abstract National Conference of the Hospital Infection Society, Liverpool, November). *Journal of Hospital Infection*, 76(S16): 0195–6701.

Hughes, J., Jennings, L. and Smith, K. (2011b) An audit of MRSA prevalence in a mental health trust. North West Research and Audit Conference, Liverpool, November.

Hughes, L. (2010) Cannabis use and psychosis. In P. Phillip, O. McKeown and T. Sandford (eds), *Dual Diagnosis: Practice in Context*. Oxford: Wiley-Blackwell.

Hunter, J. and Rawlings-Anderson, K. (2008) Respiratory assessment. *Nursing Standard*, 22: 41–3.

Hussein-Rassool, G. (2010) *Addiction for Nurses*. Oxford: Wiley-Blackwell.

Hyland, B., Judd, F., Davidson, S., Jolly, D. and Hocking, B. (2003) Case managers' attitudes to the physical health of their patients. *Australian and New Zealand Journal of Psychiatry*, 37(6): 710–14.

Infection Control Nurses' Association (2002) *Protective Clothing: Principles and Guidance*. Bathgate: Fitwise.

Iwasaki, Y., Coyle, C.P. and Shank, J.W. (2010) Leisure as a context for active living, recovery, health and life quality for persons with mental illness in a global context. *Health Promotion International*, 25(4): 483–94.

Johnson, A.M., Mercer, C.H. and Erens, B. (2002) Sexual behaviour in Britain: partnerships, practices and HIV risk behaviours. *Lancet*, 358: 1835–42.

Johnson, J.L., Moffat, B.M. and Malchy, L.A. (2010) In the shadow of a new smoke free policy: a discourse analysis of health care providers' engagement in tobacco control in community mental health. *International Journal of Mental Health Systems*, 4 (article 23).

Johnson, K. and Rawlings-Anderson, K. (2007) *Oxford Handbook of Cardiac Nursing*. Oxford: Oxford University Press.

Joint British Societies (British Cardiac Society, British Hypertension Society, Diabetes UK, HEART UK, Primary Care Cardiovascular Society, The Stroke Association) (2005) JBS 2: Joint British Societies' guidelines on prevention of cardiovascular disease in clinical practice. *Heart*, 91(Suppl V): v1–v52 (www.heartjnl.com, accessed January 2006).

Jones, A. and Jones, M. (2005) Mental health nurse prescribing: issues for the UK. *Journal of Psychiatric and Mental Health Nursing*, 12: 527–35.

Jones, F.R. (2004) Can expert patients be created? In Royal Pharmaceutical Society of Great Britain (eds) *Perspectives on the expert patient. Presentations from a seminar held at the Royal Pharmaceutical Society of Great Britain on 19 May 2003* : London: Royal Pharmaceutical Society of Great Britain.

Jones, S., Howard, L. and Thornicroft, G. (2008) 'Diagnostic overshadowing': worse physical health care for people with mental illness. *Acta Psychiatrica Scandinavica*, 118: 169–71.

Jowett, N.I. and Thompson, D.R. (2007) *Comprehensive Coronary Care*. Edinburgh: Bailliere Tindall Elsevier.

Kane, J.M., Woerner, M. and Lieberman, J. (1988) Tardive dyskinesia: prevalence, incidence, and risk factors. *Journal of Clinical Psychopharmacology*, 8(4 Suppl): 52S–56S.

Kelly, C. and McCreadie, R. (2000) Cigarette smoking and schizophrenia. *Advances in Psychiatric Treatment*, 6: 327–32.

Killian, J.G., Kerr, K., Lawrence, C. and Celermajer, D.S. (1999) Myocarditis and cardiomyopathy associated with clozapine. *Lancet*, 354: 1841–45.

Kilpatrick, C., Prieto, J. and Wigglesworth, N. (2008) Single room isolation to prevent transmission of infection: development of a patient journey tool to support safe practice. *British Journal of Infection Control*, 9(6): 19–25.

Kisely, S., Sadek, J., MacKenzie, A., Lawrence, D. and Campbell, L.A. (2008) Excess cancer mortality in psychiatric patients. *The Canadian Journal of Psychiatry*, 53(11): 753–60.

Knol, L.L., Pritchett, K. and Dunkin, J. (2010) Institutional policy changes aimed at addressing obesity among mental health clients. *Preventing Chronic Disease*, 7(3): A63. Available at: www.cdc.gov/pcd/issues/2010/may/09_0138.htm (accessed 17 July 2012).

Knol, M.J., Twisk, J.W.R, Beekman, A.T.F., Heine, R.J., Snoeke, F.J. and Pouwer, F. (2006) Depression as a risk factor for the onset of type 2 diabetes mellitus: a meta-analysis. *Diabetologica*, 49: 837–45.

Kouki, R., Schwab, U., Hassinen, M., Komulainen, P., Heikkila, H., Lakka, T.A. and Rauramaa, R. (2011) Food consumption, nutrient intake and the risk of having metabolic syndrome: the DR's EXTRA Study. *European Journal of Clinical Nutrition*, 65: 368–77.

Krentz, A.J. and Bailey, C.J. (2001) *Type 2 Diabetes in Practice*. London: The Royal Society of Medicine Press.

Lambert, T.J.R., Velakoulis, D. and Pantelis, C. (2003) Medical co-morbidity in schizophrenia. *Medical Journal of Australia*, 178: 67–70.

Lansdown, A. B. (2004) Nutrition 1; a vital consideration in the management of skin wounds. *British Journal of Nursing*, 13: S22–S28.

Laursen, T.M., Munk-Olsen, T., Agerbo, E., Gasse, C. and Mortensen, P.B. (2009) Somatic hospital contacts, invasive cardiac procedures, and mortality from heart disease in patients with severe mental disorder. *Archives of General Psychiatry*, 66(7): 713–20.

Lawn, S.J., Pols, R.G. and Barber, J.G. (2002) Smoking and quitting: a qualitative study with community psychiatric clients. *Social Science and Medicine*, 54(1): 93–104.

Lawrence, D. and Kisley, S. (2010) Inequalities in healthcare provision for people with severe mental illness. *Journal of Psychopharmacology*, 24(11): 61–8.

Lawrence, J. and May D. (2003) *Infection Control in the Community*. Edinburgh: Churchill Livingstone.

Leggett, V. and Williams, H. (2000) Bum bags and communion cups: infection control in mental health care. *Continuing Professional Development*, 2(1): 18–22.

Lemieux, J., Maunsell, E. and Provencher, L. (2008) Chemotherapy-induced alopecia and effects on quality of life among women with breast cancer: a literature review. *Psycho-Oncology*, 17: 317–28.

Leucht, S., Burkard, T., Henderson, J., Maj, M. and Sartorius, N. (2007) Physical illness and schizophrenia: a review of the literature. *Acta Psychiatrica Scandinavica*, 116: 317–33.

Lichtermann, D., Ekelund, J., Pukkala, E. and Tanskanen Lonnqvist, J. (2001) Incidence of cancer amongst persons with schizophrenia and their relatives. *Archives of General Psychiatry*, 58: 573–8.

Linden, M., Lecrubier, Y., Bellantuono, C., Benkert, O., Kisely, S. and Simon, G. (1999) The prescribing of psychotropic drugs by primary care physicians: an international collaborative study. *Journal of Clinical Psychopharmacology*, 19(2): 132–40.

Lindsay, G. and Gaw, A. (2004) *Coronary Heart Disease Prevention: A Handbook for the Healthcare Team*, Second Edition. London: Churchill Livingstone.

Lo, C., Li, M. and Rodin, G. (2008) The assessment and treatment of distress in cancer patients: overview and future directions. *Minerva Psichiatrica*, 49(2): 129–43.

Lund, B.C., Perry, P.J., Brooks, J.M. and Arndt, S. (2001) Clozapine use in patients with schizophrenia and the risk of diabetes, hyperlipidaemia and hypertension: a claims-based approach. *Archive of General Psychiatry*, 58: 1172–6.

Mackenzie, L., James, I.A., Smith, K., Barnard, D. and Robinson, D. (2008) Assessing hand hygiene in older people's care settings. *Nursing Times*, 104(32): 28–30.

Marmot, M. (2010) *Fair Society, Healthy Lives: Strategic Review of Health Inequalities in England*. London: University College London.

Matevosyan, N.R. (2009) Reproductive health in women with serious mental illness: a review. *Sex Disability*, 27: 109–18.

McAllister, J. (2004) An overview of the current asthma disease management guidance. *British Journal of Nursing*, 13: 512–17.

McCann, E. (2003) Exploring sexual and relationship possibilities for people with psychosis: a review of the literature. *Journal of Psychiatric and Mental Health Nursing*, 10: 640–49.

McCloughen, A. (2003) The association between schizophrenia and cigarette smoking: a review of the literature and implications for mental health nursing practice. *International Journal of Mental Health Nursing*, 12: 119–29.

McCloughen, A. and Foster, K. (2011) Weight gain associated with taking psychotropic medication: an integrative review. *International Journal of Mental Health Nursing*, 20: 202–22.

McCreadie, R.G. (2003) Diet, smoking and cardiovascular risk in people with schizophrenia: descriptive study. *British Journal of Psychiatry*, 183: 534–53.

McCreadie, R.G., Thara, R., Srinivasan, T.N. and Padmavathi, R. (2003) Spontaneous dyskinesia in first-degree relatives of chronically ill, never-treated people with schizophrenia. *British Journal of Psychiatry*, 183: 45–9.

McEvoy, J.P., Meyer, J.M. and Goff, D.C. et al. (2005) Prevalence of the metabolic syndrome in patients with schizophrenia: baseline results from the clinical antipsychotic trials of national estimates from NHANES III. *Schizophrenia Research*, 80: 19–32.

McIntyre, R.S., Soczynska, J.K. and Beyer, J.L. (2007) Medical comorbidity in bipolar disorder: prioritizing unmet needs. *Current Opinion in Psychiatry*, 20(4): 406–16.

McKenzie, K., Whitley, R. and Weich, S. (2002) Social capital and mental health. *British Journal of Psychiatry*, 181: 280–283.

McKeown, O. (2010) Definition, recognition and assessment. In P. Phillips, O. McKeown and T. Sandford (eds), *Dual Diagnosis: Practice in Context*. Oxford: Wiley-Blackwell.

McNally, L. and The London Development Centre (2009) *Quitting in Mind: A Guide to Implementing Stop Smoking Support in Mental Health Settings. 4.1 Pharmacological Treatment Dimensions Pharmacotherapy*. London: London Development Centre.

McNeil, A. (2001) *Smoking and Mental Health: a literature Review*. London: Action on Smoking and Health (www.ash.org).

Mears, A., Clancy, C., Banerjee, S., Crome, I. and Agbo-Quaye, S. (2001) *Co-existing Problems of Mental Disorder and Substance Misuse (Dual Diagnosis): A Training Needs Analysis*. Final Report to the Department of Health. London: Department of Health.

Meddings, S. and Perkins, R. (2002) What getting better means to staff and users of rehabilitation service: an exploratory study. *Journal of Mental Health*, 11(3): 319–25.

Meltzer, H., Lader, D., Corbin, T., Singleton, N., Jenkins, R. and Brugha, T. (2002) *Non-Fatal Suicidal Behaviour among Adults aged 16 to 74 in Great Britain*. London: The Stationery Office.

Miller, D., Caroff, S.N., Davis, S.M., Rosenheck, R.A., McEvoy, J.P., Saltz, B.L., Riggio, S., Chakos, M.H., Swartz, M.S., Keefe, R.S., Stroup, T.S. and Lieberman, J.A. (2008) Extrapyramidal side-effects of antipsychotics in a randomised trial. *British Journal of Psychiatry*, 193(4): 279–88.

Miller, W. and Rollnick, S. (2002) *Motivational Interviewing: Preparing People to Change*. New York: Guilford Press.

Ministry of Health and the New Zealand Cancer Control Trust (2003) *The New Zealand Cancer Control Strategy*. Wellington: Ministry of Health.

Morris, C. (2006) Wound management and dressing selection. *Wound Essentials*,1: 178–83.

Morrison, K.N. and Naegle, M.A. (2010) An evidence-based protocol for smoking cessation for persons with psychotic disorders. *Journal of Addictions Nursing*, 21: 79–86.

Mortensen, P.B. (1994) The occurrence of cancer in first-admitted schizophrenia patients. *Schizophrenia Research*, 12: 185–94.

Mueser, K.T., Meyer, P.S., Penn, D.L., Clancy, R., Clancy, D.M. and Salyers, M.P. (2006) The Illness Management and Recovery Program: rationale, development, and preliminary findings. *Schizophrenia Bulletin*, 32(S1): S32–S43.

Mueser, K.T., Noordsy, D.L., Drake, R.E. and Fox, L. (2003) *Integrated Treatment for Dual Disorders: A Guide to Effective Practice*. New York: Guilford.

Munday, D., Dale, J. and Murray, S. (2007) Choice and place of death: individual preferences, uncertainty, and the availability of care. *Journal of the Royal Society of Medicine*, 100(5): 211–15.

Munetz, M.R. and Benjamin, S. (1988) How to examine patients using the Abnormal Involuntary Movement Scale. *Hospital and Community Psychiatry*, 39(11): 1172–7.

Muntoni, S. and Muntoni, S. (2011) Insulin resistance: pathophysiology and rationale for treatment. *Annals of Nutrition and Metabolism*, 58: 25–36.

Murdoch, S. (1992) A safe environment for care: infection control nurses' role in mental health units. *Professional Nurse*, 7(8): 519–22.

Murdoch, S. and Cowell, F. (1993) Sharp shocks. *Nursing Times*, 89(2): 64–8.

Murray, S.A., Kendall, M., Boyd, K. and Sheikh, S. (2005) Illness trajectories and palliative care. *British Medical Journal*, 330: 1007–11.

Nash, M. (2005) Physical care skills: a training needs analysis of impatient and community mental health nurses. *Mental Health Practice*, 9(4): 20–23.

Nash, M. (2010a) *Physical Health and Wellbeing in Mental Health Nursing*. Maidenhead: McGraw-Hill.

Nash, M. (2010b) Mental health nurses' diabetes care skills – a training needs analysis. *British Journal of Nursing*, 18(16): 626–30.

National Cancer Peer Review–National Cancer Action Team (2010) *National Cancer Peer Review Programme. Manual for Cancer Services: Psychological Support Measures*. London: National Health Service.

National Health Service and the University of Nottingham (2008) *Advance Care Planning: A Guide for Health and Care Staff*. London: Department of Health.

National Health Service Information Center (2010) *Statistics on Smoking: England*. Available at: www.ic/nhs.uk/statistics.

National Health Service Information Centre (2011) *Quarterly Analysis of Mental Capacity Act 2005: Deprivation of Liberty Safeguards Assessments England*. London: Department of Health.

National Institute for Health and Clinical Excellence (2002) *Core Interventions in the Treatment and Management of Schizophrenia in Primary and Secondary Care (Clinical Guideline 1)*. London: NICE.

National Institute for Health and Clinical Excellence (2004a) *Multifactorial Falls Risk Assessment*. London: NICE.

National Institute for Health and Clinical Excellence (2004b) *Self-harm: The Short-term Physical and Psychological Management and Secondary Prevention of Self-Harm in Primary and Secondary Care*. London: NICE.

National Institute for Health and Clinical Excellence (2005) *Pressure Ulcers: The Management of Pressure Ulcers in Primary and Secondary Care*. London: NICE.

National Institute for Health and Clinical Excellence (2006a) *The Management of Bipolar Disorder in Adults, Children and Adolescents, in Primary and Secondary Care*. London: NICE.

National Institute for Health and Clinical Excellence (2006b) *Type 2 Diabetes – Obesity*. London: NICE.

National Institute for Health and Clinical Excellence (2006c) *Nutrition Support in Adults*. London: NICE.

National Institute for Health and Clinical Excellence (2006d) *Hypertension: management of hypertension in adults in primary care*. London: National Institute for Health and Clinical Excellence.

National Institute for Health and Clinical Excellence (2007) *Antenatal and Postnatal Mental Health*. London: NICE.

National Institute for Health and Clinical Excellence (2008) *Smoking Cessation Services in Primary Care, Pharmacies, Local Authorities and Workplaces, Particularly for Manual Working Groups, Pregnant Women and Hard-to-reach Communities*. London: NICE.

National Institute for Health and Clinical Excellence (2009) *Schizophrenia: Core Interventions in the Treatment and Management of Schizophrenia in Adults in Primary and Secondary Care* (Updated edition). London: NICE.

National Institute for Health and Clinical Excellence (2010a) *Chronic Obstructive Pulmonary Disease: Management of Chronic Obstructive Pulmonary Disease in Adults in Primary and Secondary Care*. London: NICE.

National Institute for Health and Clinical Excellence (2010b) *Alcohol-use Disorders: Diagnosis and Clinical Management of Alcohol-related Physical Complications*. London: NICE.

National Institute for Health and Clinical Excellence (2010c) *Psychosis with Coexisting Substance Misuse: Assessment and Management in Adults and Young People*. London: NICE.

National Institute for Health and Clinical Excellence (2011a) *Type 2 Diabetes – Newer Agents: Short Guidance.* London: NICE.

National Institute for Health and Clinical Excellence (2011b) *Tuberculosis: Clinical Diagnosis and Management of Tuberculosis and Measures for its Prevention and Control.* London: NICE.

National Institute for Health and Clinical Excellence and the National Collaboration Centre for Primary Care (2006)*Obesity: The Prevention, Identification, Assessment and Management of Overweight and Obesity in Adults and Children.*London: NICE

National Patient Safety Agency (2005) *Clean Your Hands Campaign.* London: National Patient Safety Agency.

National Patient Safety Agency (2008) *NPSA Alert: Clean Hands Safe Lives.* London: National Patient Safety Agency.

National Prescribing Service (2011) RADAR (Rational Assessment of Drugs and Research) *Varenicline (Champix) for Smoking Cessation.* Australia: National Prescribing Service. Available at: www.nps.org.au/health_professionals/publications/nps_radar/2011/april_2011/varenicline (accessed 2 March 2012).

National Treatment Agency (2008) *Harm Reduction Strategy – Guidance to Support Adult Drug Treatment Planning 2009/2010.* London: National Treatment Agency for Substance Misuse.

Newcomer, J.W., Haupt, D.W., Fucetola, R., Melson, A.K., Schweiger, J.A., Cooper, B.P. and Selke, G. (2002) Abnormalities in glucose regulation during antipsychotic treatment of schizophrenia. *Archives of General Psychiatry*, 59: 337–45.

Newman, S.C. and Bland, R.C. (1991) Mortality in a cohort of patients with schizophrenia: a record lineage study. *Canadian Journal of Psychiatry*, 36: 293–45.

Nimwegen, L.J., Storosum, J.G., Blumer, R.M., Allick, G., Venema, H.W., de Haan, L., Becker, H., van Amelsvoort, T., Ackermans, M.T., Fliers, E., Serlie, M.J. and Sauerwein, H.P. (2008) Hepatic insulin resistance in antipsychotic naive patients with schizophrenia: a detailed study of glucose metabolism with stable isotopes. *Journal of Clinical Endocrinology and Metabolism*, 93: 572–7.

Nisell, M., Nomikos, G.G. and Svensson, T.H. (2009) Nicotine dependence, midbrain dopamine systems and psychiatric disorders. *Basic and Clinical Pharmacology and Toxicology*, 76: 157–2.

Northrop, M. (2009) Physical health issues in mental health practice. In N. Wrycraft (ed.), *An Introduction to Mental Health Nursing.* Maidenhead: McGraw-Hill.

Nursing and Midwifery Council (2010) *Standards for Pre-registration Nursing Education.* London: NMC.

O'Connor, S. (2008) Surgery. In J. Corner and C. Bailey (eds), *Cancer Nursing: Care in Context*, 2nd edn. Oxford: Blackwell.

O'Sullivan, J., Gilbert, J. and Ward, W. (2006) Addressing the health and lifestyle issues of people with a mental illness: the healthy living programme. *Australian Psychiatry*, 14(2): 150–55.

Office of Health Economics (2009) *OHE Compendium of Health Statistics.* Available at: www.ohecompendium.org/ (accessed 10 November 2010).

Orchard, T.J., Temprosa, M., Goldberg, R., Haffner, S., Ratner, R., Marcovina, S., and Fowler, S. (2005) The effect of metformin and intensive lifestyle intervention on the metabolic syndrome: the Diabetes Prevention Program randomized trial. *Annals of International Medicine*, 142(8) (19 April): 611–19.

Osborn, D.P.J., King, M.B. and Nazareth, I. (2003) Participation in screening for cardiovascular risk by people with schizophrenia or similar mental illnesses: cross sectional study in general practice. *British Medical Journal*, 326: 1122–3.

Osborn, P.J., Levy, G., Nazareth, I., Petersen, I., Islam, A. and King, M.B. (2007) Relative risk of cardiovascular and cancer mortality in people with severe mental illness from the United Kingdom's general practice research database. *Archives of General Psychiatry*, 64: 242–9.

Osby, U., Correia, N., Brant, L., Ekbom, A. and Sparen, P. (2000) Mortality and cause of death in schizophrenia in Stockholm County, Sweden. *Schizophrenia Research*, 45: 21–8.

Osher, F.C. and Kofoed, L.L. (1989) Treatment of patients with psychiatric and psychoactive substance abuse disorders. *Hospital and Community Psychiatry*, 40: 1025–30.

Ott, M. and French, R. (2009) Hand hygiene compliance among health care staff and student nurses in a mental health setting. *Issues in Mental Health Nursing*, 30: 702–4.

Oud, M.J.T., Schuling, J., Slooff, C.J., Groenier, K.H., Dekker, J.H. and Meyboom-de Jong, B. (2009) Care for patients with severe mental illness: the general practitioner's role perspective. *BMC Family Practice*, 10:29 doi: 10.1186/1471-2296-10-29.

Ousey, K. and Ousey, C. (2010) Intervention strategies for people who self-harm. *Wound UK*, 6(4): 34–40.

Pal, S.K., Katheria, V. and Hurria, A. (2010) Evaluating the older patient with cancer: understanding frailty and the geriatric assessment. *CA: A Cancer Journal for Clinicians*, 60(2): 120–32.

Pan, A., Lucas, M., Sun, Q., van Dam, R.M., Franco, O.H., Willet, W.C., Mason, J.E., Rexrode, K.M., Ascheio, A. and Hu, F.B. (2011) Increased mortality risk in women with depression and diabetes. *Archives of General Psychiatry*, 68(1): 42–50.

Papageorgiou, A., King, M., Janmohamed, A., Davidson, O. and Dawson, J. (2002) Advance directives for patients compulsorily admitted to hospital with serious mental illness. *British Journal of Psychiatry*, 181: 513–19.

Parks, J., Svensden, D., Singer, P. and Foti, M.E. (2006) *Morbidity and Mortality in People with Serious Mental Illness*. Alexandria, VA: National Association of State Mental Health Program Directors.

Peacock, S. (2004) Systematic health assessment: a case study. *Practice Nursing*, 15(6): 270–74.

Peate, I. (2005) *Manual of Sexually Transmitted Infections*. London: Whurr.

Perkins, L. (2000) Nutritional balance in wound healing, *Clinical Nutrition Update*, 1 (5): 8–10.

Perry, C. (2007) *Essential Skills for Nurses: Infection Prevention and Control*. Oxford: Blackwell.

Phelan, M., Stradins, L. and Morrison, S. (2001) Physical health of people with severe mental illness. *British Medical Journal*, 322: 443–4.

Phelan, M., Stradins, L., Amin, D., Isadore, R., Hitrov, C., Doyle, A. and Inglis, R. (2004) The Physical Health Check: a tool for mental health workers. *Journal of Mental Health*, 13(3): 277–84.

Praharaj, S.K., Jana, A.K., Goyal, N. and Sinha, V.K. (2011) Metformin for olanzapine-induced weight gain: a systematic review and meta-analysis. *British Journal of Clinical Pharmacology*, 71(3): 377–82.

Pratt, R.P., Pellowe, C.M., Wilson, J.A., Loveday, H.P., Harper, P.J., Jones, S.R.L.S., McDougall, C. and Wilcox, M.H. (2007) Epic 2: National Evidence-Based Guidelines for Preventing Healthcare-Associated Infections in Hospitals in England. *Journal of Hospital Infection*, 65 (Suppl.): S1–S64.

Prochaska, J.O. and DiClemente C.C. (1986) Towards a comprehensive model of change. In U. Miller and N. Heather (eds), *Treating Addictive Behaviors*. New York: Plenum Press.

Quinn, C. and Browne, G. (2009) Sexuality of people living with mental illness: a collaborative challenge for mental health nurses. *International Journal of Mental Health Nursing*, 18: 195–203.

Raphael, T. and Parsons, J.P. (1921) Blood sugar studies in dementia praecox and manic-depressive insanity. *Archives of Neurology and Psychiatry*, 5: 587–709.

Rasmor, M. and Brown, C.M. (2003) Physical examination for the occupational health nurse. *AAOHN [American Association of Occupational Health Nurses] Journal*, 51(9): 390–403.

Ratschen, E., Britton, J. and McNeill, A. (2011) The smoking culture in psychiatry: time for change. *British Journal of Psychiatry*, 198: 6–7.

Reaven, G.M. (1995) Pathophysiology of insulin resistance in human disease. *Physiological Reviews*, 75: 473–86.

Regier, D., Farmer, M.E., Rae, D.S., Locke, B.Z., Keith, B.J., Judd, L.L. and Godwin, F.K. (1990) Co-morbidity of mental disorders with alcohol and other drug abuse: results from the epidemiological catchment area (ECA) study. *Journal of the American Medical Association*, 264: 2511–18.

Richardson, C.R. and Faulkner, G. (2005) Integrating physical activity into mental health services for persons with serious mental illness. *Psychiatric Services*, 56(3): 324–31.

Richens, J. (2004) Main presentations of sexually transmitted infections in male patients. In M. Adler, F. Cowan, P. French, H. Mitchell and J. Richens (eds), *ABC of Sexually Transmitted Infections*, 5th edn. London: BMJ Books.

Roberts, L., Roalfe, A., Wilson, S. and Lester, H. (2007) Physical health care of patients with schizophrenia in primary care: a comparative study. *Family Practice*, 24: 34–40.

Roberts, S.H. and Bailey, J.E. (2011) Incentives and barriers to lifestyle interventions for people with severe mental illness: a narrative synthesis of quantitative, qualitative and mixed methods of studies. *Journal of Advanced* Nursing, 67(4): 690–708.

Robson, D. and Gray, R. (2007) Serious mental illness and physical health problems: a discussion paper. *International Journal of Nursing Studies*, 44: 457–66.

Robson, D. and Gray, R. (2009) Physical healthcare and serious mental illness. In I. Norman and I. Ryrie (eds), *The Art and Science of Mental Health Nursing*, 2nd edition. Maidenhead: McGraw-Hill.

Rosenberg, S.D., Goodman, L.A., Osher, F.C., Swartz, M.S., Essock, S.M. et al. (2001) Prevalence of HIV, hepatitis B and hepatitis C in people with severe mental illness. *American Journal of Public Health*, 91(1): 31–7.

Rowe, C., Bannerman, M. and Church, N. (2009) Health promotion. In K. French (ed.), *Sexual Health*. Oxford: Wiley-Blackwell.

Royal College of General Practitioners and Royal College of Psychiatry (2008) *Primary Care Guidance on Smoking and Mental Health*. RCGP & RCPSYCH Forum: working together for mental wellbeing). London: RCGP and RCPSYCH. Available at: www.mentalhealth.org.uk/publications/smoking-mental-health-primary-care/ (accessed 5 March 2012).

Royal College of Psychiatrists (2009) *Physical Health in Mental Health*. Occasional Paper 67 – Final Report of a Scoping Group. London: Royal College of Psychiatrists.

Ruidavets, J.B., Bongard, V., Dallongeville, J., Arveiler, D., Ducimetière, P., Perret, B., Simon, C., Amouyel, P. and Ferrières, J. (2007) High consumptions of grains, fish, dairy products and combinations of these are associated with a low prevalence of metabolic syndrome. *Journal of Epidemiology and Community Health*, 61: 810–17.

Rushforth, H., Warner, J., Burge, D. and Glasper, E.A. (1998) Nursing physical assessment skills: implications for UK practice. *British Journal of Nursing*, 7(16): 965–70.

Russell, L. (2002) Understanding physiology of wound healing and how dressings help. In R. White (ed.), *Trends in Wound Care*. British Journal of Nursing Monograph. London: Quay Books.

Saha, S., Chant, D. and McGrath, J. (2007) Systematic review of mortality in schizophrenia: is the differential mortality gap worsening over time? *Archives of General Psychiatry*, 64(10): 1123–31.

Savulescu, J. (2007) Autonomy, the good life and controversial choices. In R. Rhodes, L.P. Francis and A. Silvers (eds), *The Blackwell Guide to Medical Ethics*. Oxford: Blackwell.

Scarborough, P., Wickramasinghe, K., Bhatnagar, P. and Rayner, M. (2011) Trends in coronary heart disease 1961–2011, British Heart Foundation Health Promotion Research Group, Department of Public Health, University of Oxford.

Schmitz, N., Wang, J., Ashok, M. and Alain, L. (2009) The impact of psychological distress on functional disability in asthma: results from the Canadian community health survey, *Psychosomatics*, 50 (1): 42–9.

Schmutte, T., Flanagan, E., Bedregal, L., Ridgway, P., Sells, D., Styron, T. and Davidson, L. (2009) Self-efficacy and self-care: missing ingredients in health and healthcare among adults with serious mental illnesses. *Psychiatric Quarterly*, 80: 1–8.

Scott, K.M., Oakley Browne, M.A., McGee, M.A. and Wells, J.E. (2006) Mental-physical comorbidity in Te Rau Hinengaro: The New Zealand mental health survey. *Australian and New Zealand Journal of Psychiatry*, 40 (10): 882–8.

Sears, M.R. (2008) The definition and diagnosis of asthma. *Allergy*, 48: 12–16.

Seedhouse, D. (2001) *Health: The Foundations for Achievement*. Chichester, UK: John Wiley & Sons.

Seeman, M.V. (2011) Preventing breast cancer in women with schizophrenia. *Acta Psychiatrica Scandinavica*, 123(2): 107–17.

Seidel, H., Ball, J., Dains, J. and Benedict, G.W. (2003) *Mosby's Guide to Physical Examination*, 5th edn. St Louis, MO: Mosby.

Sepulveda, C., Marlin, A., Yoshida, T. and Ullrich, A. (2002) Palliative care: The World Health Organization's global perspective. *Journal of Pain and Symptom Management*, 24 (2): 91–6.

Shakher, J. and Barnett, A.H. (2004) Diabetes, obesity and cardiovascular disease: therapeutic implications. In H. Barnett and S. Kumar (eds), *Obesity and Diabetes*. Chichester, UK: John Wiley & Sons.

Shiner, B., Whitley, B., Van Citters, A.D., Pratt, S.I. and Bartels, S.J. (2008) Learning what matters for patients: qualitative evaluation of a health promotion program for those with serious mental illness. *Health Promotion International*, 23(3): 275–82.

Shuel, F., White, F., Jones, M. and Grey, R. (2010) Using the serious mental illness health improvement profile (HIP) to identify physical problems in a cohort of community patients: a pragmatic case study. *International Journal of Nursing Studies*, 47: 136–45.

Siegel, J.D., Rhineheart, E., Jackson, M. and Chiarello, L. (2007) 2007 *Guideline for Isolation Precautions: Preventing Transmission of Infectious Agents in Healthcare Settings*. Atlanta, GA: The Healthcare Infection Control Practices Advisory Committee. Available at: www.cdc.gov/ncidod/dhqp/pdf/guidelines/isolation2007.pdf (accessed 4 February 2012).

Silvestri, L., Sarginson, R.E., Hughes, J., Milanese, M., Gregori, D. and van Saene, H.K.F. (2002) Most nosocomial pneumonias are not due to nosocomial bacteria in ventilated patients: evaluation of the accuracy of the 48hour time cut-off using carriage as gold standard. *Anaesthesia and Intensive Care*, 30: 275–82.

Simonelli-Munoz, A.J., Fortea, M.I., Salorio, P., Gallego-Gomez, J.I., Sanchez-Bautista, S. and Balanza, S. (2012) Dietary habits of patients with schizophrenia: a self-reported questionnaire survey. *International Journal of Mental Health Nursing*, 21: 220–28.

Simpson, G.M. and Angus, J.W.S. (1970) A rating scale for extrapyramidal side effects. *Acta Psychiatrica Scandinavica*, 4 (S212): 11–19.

Singh, I., Sandhu, S. and Kaur, B. (2010) *Secondary Sexual Dysfunction and Antipsychotics: A Survey of Psychiatrists in Greater Manchester.* Available at: http://priory.com/psychiatry/sexual_side_effects.htm (accessed 3 February 2012).

Slovacek, L., Slovackova, B., Slanska, I., Petera, J., Priester, P., Filip, S. and Kopecky, J. (2009) Depression symptoms and health-related quality of life among patients with metastatic breast cancer in programme of palliative cancer care. *Neoplasma*, 56(6): 467–72.

Sokal, J., Messias, E., Dickerson, F.B., Kreyenbuhl, J., Brown, C.H., Goldberg, R.W. and Dixon, L.B. (2004) Comorbidity of medical illness among adults with serious mental illness who are receiving community psychiatric services. *Journal of Nervous & Mental Disease*, 192: 421–7.

Sorrentino, M.J. (2011) The metabolic syndrome. In M.J. Sorrentino (ed.), *Hyperlipidaemia in Primary Care: A Practical Guide to Risk Reduction.* New York: Humana Press.

Soundy, A., Faulkner, G. and Taylor, A. (2007) Exploring variability and perceptions of lifestyle physical activity among individuals with severe and enduring mental health problems: a qualitative study. *Journal of Mental Health*, 16: 493–503.

Stenton, C. (2008) The MRC Breathlessness Scale. *Occupational Medicine*, 58(3): 226–7.

Stokes, C. (2003) Dietary sugar intake and the severity of symptoms of schizophrenia. MSc Thesis. Sheffield: University of Sheffield.

Strassnig, M., Singh Brar, J. and Ganguli, R. (2003) Nutritional assessment of patients with schizophrenia. *Schizophrenia Bulletin*, 29(2): 393–7.

Sukanta, S., Chant, D. and McGrath, J. (2007) A systematic review of mortality in schizophrenia: is the differential mortality gap worsening over time? *Archive of General Psychiatry*, 64(10): 1123–31.

Swanson, J.W., Swartz, M.S., Elbogen, E.B., Van Dorn, R.A., Ferron, J., Wagner, H.R., McCauley, B.J. and Kim, M. (2006) Facilitated psychiatric advance directives: a randomised control trial of an intervention to foster advance treatment planning among persons with severe mental illness. *American Journal of Psychiatry*, 163: 1943–51.

Swett, C. (1975) Drug-induced dystonia. *American Journal of Psychiatry*, 132(5): 532–4.

Taylor, L. (1978) An evaluation of handwashing techniques. *Nursing Times*, 74: 108–11.

Taylor, T.T., Hawton, K., Fortune, S. and Kapur, N. (2009) Attitudes towards clinical services among people who self-harm: a systematic review. *British Journal of Psychiatry*, 194: 104–10.

Thirlaway, K. and Upton, D. (2009) *The Psychology of Lifestyle: Promoting Healthy Behaviour.* London: Routledge.

Thomas, S. (1997) A structured approach to the selection of dressings. *World Wide Wounds* [Online], www.worldwidewounds.com/1997/july/Thomas-Guide/Dress-Select.html (accessed 9 January 2012).

Thompson, I.E., Melia, K.M., Boyd, K.M. and Horsburgh, D. (2006) *Nursing Ethics*, 5th edn. Edinburgh and London: Churchill Livingstone.

Tiihonen, J., Lönnqvist, J., Wahlbeck, K., Klaukka, T., Niskanen, L., Tanskanen, A. and Haukka J. (2009) An 11-year follow-up of mortality in patients with schizophrenia: a population-based cohort study. FIN11 Study. *The Lancet*, 374: 620–27.

Timmons, J. (2005) *Essential Wound Management: An Introduction for Undergraduates.* London: Wounds UK.

Tobias, J. and Hochhauser, D. (2010) *Cancer and Its Management*, 6th edn. Oxford: Wiley-Blackwell.

Tortora, G.J. and Grabowski, S.J. (2003) *Principles of Anatomy and Physiology.* New York: John Wiley.

Tosh, G., Clifton, A. and Bachner, M. (2011) General physical health advice for people with serious mental illness. *Schizophrenia Bulletin*, 37(4): 671–3. *Cochrane Database of Systematic Reviews*, Issue 2: CD008567. The Cochrane Collaboration, published by John Wiley & Sons, Ltd.

Tosh, G., Clifton, A., Mala, S. et al. (2010) Physical health monitoring for people with serious mental illness. *Cochrane Database of Systematic Reviews*, 17(3): CD008298. The Cochrane Collaboration, published by John Wiley & Sons, Ltd.

Tschoner, A., Engl, J., Rettenbacher, M., Edlinger, M., Kaser, S., Tatarczyk, T., Effenberger, M., Patsch, J.R., Fleischhacker, W.W. and Ebenbichler, C.F. (2009) Effects of six second generation antipsychotics on body weight and metabolism: risk assessment and results from a prospective study. *Pharmacopsychiatry*, 42(1): 29–34.

University of Manchester (2006) *Five Year Report by the National Confidential Inquiry into Suicide and Homicide with People with Mental Illness*. Manchester: University of Manchester.

Ussher, M., Stanbury, L., Cheeseman, V. and Faulkner, G. (2007) Physical activity preferences and perceived barriers to activity among persons with severe mental illness in the United Kingdom. *Psychiatric Services*, 58: 405–8.

Van Citters, A.D., Pratt, S.L., Jue, K., Williams, G., Miller, P.T., Xie, H. and Bartels, S.J. (2010) A pilot evaluation of the In SHAPE individualized health promotion intervention for adults with mental illness. *Community Mental Health Journal*, 46: 540–52.

Voderholzer, U., Dersch, R., Dickhut, H.H., Herter, A., Freyer, T. and Berger, M. (2011) Physical fitness in depressive patients and impact of illness course and disability. *Journal of Affective Disorders*, 128: 160–64.

Wakley, G., Cunnion, M. and Chambers, R. (2003) *Improving Sexual Health*. Oxford: Radcliffe Medical Press.

Waldrock, H. (2009) The essence of physical health care. In P. Callaghan, J. Playle and L. Cooper (eds), *Mental Health Nursing Skills*. Oxford: Oxford University Press.

Waldrop, J. and Doughty, D. (2000) Wound healing physiology. In R. Bryant (ed.), *Acute and Chronic Wounds: Nursing Management*, 2nd edn. St Louis, MO: Mosby.

Wallace, M. (2001) Real progress: the patient's perspective. *International Clinical Psychopharmacology*, 16 (suppl. 1): 21–4.

Wand, T. and Murray, L. (2008) Let's get physical. *International Journal of Mental Health Nursing*, 17(5): 363–9.

Warner, P.H., Rowe, T. and Whipple, B. (1999) Shedding light on sexual history. *American Journal of Nursing*, 99(6): 34–41.

Watson, D. (2008) Pneumonia: recognising signs and symptoms. *Nursing Times*, 104: 28–9.

Weaver, T., Zenobia, C.V., Carnwath, Z., Madden, P., Renton, A., Stimson, G., Tyrer, P., Barnes, T., Bench, C. and Paterson, S. (2003) Co-morbidity of substance misuse and mental illness in community mental health and substance misuse services. *British Journal of Psychiatry*, 183: 304–13.

Weber, M. (2010) The importance of exercise for individuals with chronic mental illness. *Journal of Psychosocial Nursing*, 48(10): 35–40.

Weiser, P., Becker, T., Losert, C., et al. (2009) European network for promoting the physical health of residents in psychiatric and social care facilities (HELPS): background, aims and methods. *BMC Public Health*, 9: 315. doi:10.1186/1471-2458-9-315. Available at: www.biomedcentral.com/1471-2458/9/315 (accessed 12 January 2012).

Wells, M. (2008) The impact of cancer. In J. Corner and C. Bailey (eds), *Cancer Nursing: Care in Context*, 2nd edn. Oxford: Blackwell.

Wetterling, T. (2001) Bodyweight gain with atypical antipsychotics: A comparative review. *Drug Safety*, 24: 59–73.

Wheeler, A., Harrison, J., Mohini, P., Nardan, J., Tsai, A. and Tsai, E. (2010) Cardiovascular risk assessment in mental health: whose role is it anyway? *Community Mental Health Journal*, 46(6): 531–9.

White, J., Gray, R.J., Swift, L., Barton, G.R. and Jones, M. (2011) The serious mental illness health improvement profile: study protocol for a cluster randomised control trial. *Trials*, 12: 167.

Wildgust, J.M. and Beary, M. (2010) Review: are there modifiable risk factors which will reduce the excess mortality in schizophrenia? *Journal of Psychopharmacology*, 24(11) (Suppl. 4): 37–50.

Wills, S. (2005) *Drugs of Abuse*. London: Pharmaceutical Press.

Wilson, J. (2006) *Infection Control in Clinical Practice*, 3rd edn. London: Bailliere Tindall Elsevier.

Winter, G.D. (1962) Formation of the scab and the rate of epithelialisation of superficial wounds in the young domestic pig. *Nature*, 193: 293–4.

Wirshing, D., Boyd, J., Meng, L., Ballon, J., Marder, S. and Wirshing, W. (2002) The effects of novel antipsychotics on glucose and lipid levels. *Journal of Clinical Psychiatry*, 63(10): 856–65.

Witchel, H.J., Hancox, J.C. and Nutt D.J. (2003) Psychotropic drugs, cardiac arrhythmia and sudden death. *Journal of Clinical Psychopharmacology*, 23: 58–77.

Wolkowitz, O.M., Epel, E.S., Reus, V.I. and Mellon, S.H. (2010) Depression gets old fast: do stress and depression accelerate cell aging? *Depress Anxiety*, 27: 327–38.

World Association for Sexual Health (1999) *Declaration of Sexual Rights*, adopted in Hong Kong at the 14th World Congress of Sexology.

World Health Organization (1986) *Ottawa Charter*. Geneva: WHO.

World Health Organization (1999) *Definitions, Diagnosis and Classification of Diabetes Mellitus: Report of a WHO Consultation*. Geneva: WHO.

World Health Organization (2000) *Promotion of Sexual Health: Recommendations for Action*. Geneva: WHO.

World Health Organization (2002a) *World Health Organization Strategy for the Prevention and Control of Chronic Respiratory Diseases*. Geneva: WHO.

World Health Organization (2002b) *National Cancer Control Programmes: Policies and Managerial Guidelines*, 2nd edn. Geneva: WHO.

World Health Organization (2002c) *Working Definitions – Sexual Rights*. Geneva: WHO.

World Health Organization (2003a) *Global Strategy on Diet, Physical Activity and Health*. Geneva: WHO.

World Health Organization (2003b) *Adherence to Action: Evidence for Action*. Geneva: WHO.

World Health Organization (2009) *Patient Safety: A World Alliance for Safer Health Care. WHO Guidelines on Hand Hygiene in Health Care*. First Global Patient Safety Challenge: Clean Care is Safer Care. Geneva: WHO.

World Health Organization (2011) *Global Status Report on Alcohol and Health*. Geneva: WHO.

World Health Organization (2012) *Sexual Health*. Geneva: WHO

Wounds UK (2006) *Best Practice Statement: Care of the Older Person's Skin*. London: Wounds UK. Available at: www.wounds-uk.com/pdf/content_8951.pdf (accessed 16 February 2012).

Wulsin, L.R. (2000) Does depression kill?. *Archives of Internal Medicine*, 160 (12): 1731–2.

Zimmerman, U., Kraus, T., Himmerich, H., Skuld, A. and Pollmacher, T. (2003) Epidemiology, implications and mechanisms underlying drug-induced weight gain in psychiatric patients. *Journal of Psychiatry Research*, 37: 193–220.

INDEX

Page references to Figures or Tables will be in *italics*

LIBRARY UNIVERSITY OF CHESTER

LIBRARY, UNIVERSITY OF CHESTER